SVALI

SVALI SPEAKS

BREAKING FREE OF CULT PROGRAMMING

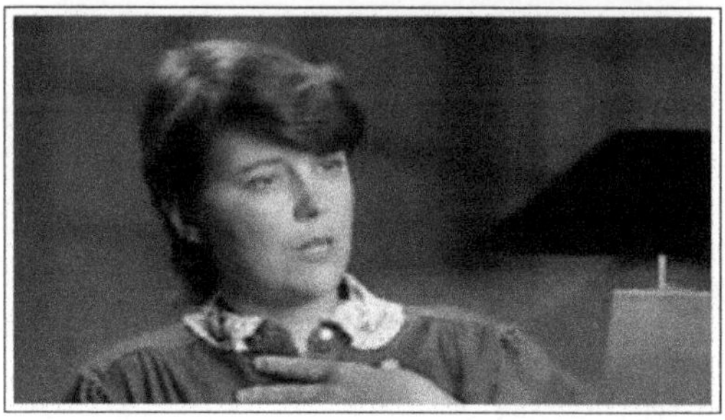

OMNIA VERITAS

SVALI

SVALI SPEAKS – BREAKING FREE OF CULT PROGRAMMING

Published by
OMNIA VERITAS LTD

OMNIA VERITAS

www.omnia-veritas.com

ABOUT THE AUTHOR

Hi, my name is Svali. Both I and my entire family were involved in a cult group until several years ago, when we broke free. I used to be a programmer in the cult, and now I want to share the knowledge that I have to help others.

It is possible to break free of cult abuse if a person is involved. It is a long, heart-breaking process, but well worth it. In the articles that I will be providing, I hope to help the survivor of cult abuse find tools to help in their journey towards freedom.

I have been a consultant to an on-line survivors group that helps people dealing with issues related to cult programming and becoming free, for the past year and a half. I myself have been in therapy for ritual abuse and DID for nine years, with the last five being aware of the recent cult abuse.

I am also a writer, and a registered nurse. I currently work as a diabetic educator in Texas 20 hours a week.

I have also self-published a book on breaking free of cult programming, which several experts in the field have said has "invaluable information" for the survivor of ritual abuse.

Both my ex-husband and my two children broke free of cult abuse last year. My children are living with me while my husband is working on healing. They all have DID (dissociative identity disorder, formerly known as multiple personality disorder) as well, which makes life at home interesting! I am currently married to my second husband, who is also a recovered DID and who got out of the cult five years ago.

EQUIPMENT FREQUENTLY USED BY TRAINERS

It may help therapists to realize the equipment that trainers use. If their client describes these items, which may appear quite sophisticated, believe them. The cult has become quite technologically advanced.

Training room: the average training room is a neutral colored room, with walls painted either a dull gray, white, or beige. Some may be painted in various colors, as part of color coding. They are often located in secret underground rooms, or basements of large private residences, and will be entered from the main building through a covered doorway. Impromptu training rooms may be set up during military exercises outdoors, in covered canvas tents.

Trainers: the Illuminati have a rule: there must always be a minimum of two trainers working with a person. This prevents a trainer from being either too severe, or permissive, or developing too close a bond with the subject; the watchful eye of the other trainer prevents this. Younger trainers are paired with older, more experienced trainers. The older trainer will teach the younger, who does most of the actual work. If the younger is unable to finish a task, or loses heart, the older one will step in.

Head trainers: will teach, they will also work with the council leaders and hierarchy. All members are required to come in for a "tune up" (reinforcing programming), even top leaders, from time to time.

EEG machine: will often have abbreviated hookups for quick use. Used extensively with brain wave programming; also to verify that a certain alter is out when called up. May be used to verify deep trance state before initiating deep programming. Trainers are taught to read these readouts.

Trainer's table: a large table, frequently steel covered with plastic, or easily cleaned material. On the sides at intervals are restraints for arms, legs, neck to prevent movement.

Trainer's chair: large chair with arm rests. Will have restraints as above at intervals to restrain movement while person sits in chair.

Shock equipment: models and types are quite varied, depending on age and company. Most have a set of rubber covered wires, with electrodes that may be connected with Velcro, rubber (steel tips imbedded under finger and toe nail beds), or gel pads (larger body areas such as chest, arms, legs). Some are tiny electrodes, which can be taped next to eyes, or placed within genitalia. These are connected to the "shock box", which has controls that can determine amount of electricity , and frequency, if interval shocks are desired.

Drugs: any number of opiates, barbiturates, hypnotics, sedatives, anesthetic agents. Resuscitative drugs, antidotes are also kept, clearly labeled and indexed. Many drugs, especially experimental ones, are only known by code names, such as "alphin 1".

CPR equipment: in case person has adverse reaction to drugs or programming. At times, a child alter will come out inadvertently during a programming sequence, and will be overdosed with the drugs meant for adult alters. The trainers must give it the antidote, and resuscitate it, just as if a real child is out. They are well aware of this fact, and will severely punish child alters, to teach them to come out only when called out.

Virtually reality headsets: the keystone in recent years. Many programming sequences utilize holographic images, and virtual reality set ups, including assassination programs, where the person realistically "kills" another human being. These virtual disks are far more advanced than those in video arcades.

Body building equipment: used in military training to increase fitness, lean body mass.

Steel instruments: used to insert into orifices, cause pain

Stretch machine: used as punishment, "stretches " person without breaking bones. Extremely painful.

Trainer's grids and projectors: used to project grids on wall or ceiling.

Movie projector: to show movies, although new VR disks are replacing these computer: collect and analyze data; keep computer grid on person's system. Current military computer access codes will be used to download into governmental computers.

Trainer's Journals: contain indexed copies of subject's systems, including key alters, command codes, etc.

Comfort objects: used to comfort subject afterwards. May be toy or candy for child alters, or oils for massage. Warm towels, or beverages may be given, as the trainer "bonds with" and comforts person they worked with. This is probably the most important part of the training process, as the trainer explains calmly, kindly how well the person did, how proud they are of them.

CHAPTER ONE

AN OVERVIEW OF THE ILLUMINATI

In order to understand Illuminati cult programming, it is first necessary to understand a bit about the structure and philosophy of the organization. The Illuminati are a group of people who follow a philosophy known as "Illuminism" or "enlightenment". The Illuminati were named several hundred years ago, but trace their roots and history to the ancient mystery religions of Egypt, ancient Babylon, and even Mesopotamia. Out of these ancient religions, which were practiced secretly over hundreds and hundreds of years, there arose esoteric groups which continued to practice the rites, traditions, and enculturation brought in from the original groups.

Over the centuries, these groups practiced openly in some countries, and covertly in countries where Christianity or other religions opposed their practices. Some of the groups which came out of these ancient roots included the order of the Knights Templar, Rosicrucian's, Baphetomism, and Druidic cults. These groups were the forerunners, or roots, of modern day Illuminism. The original Illuministic leaders chose to take what they felt were the best practices of each root religion, combine them into principles, then organized these principles according to specific guidelines.

Modern day Illuminism is a philosophy funded by the wealthy, but practiced in all social strata. It is a philosophy whose tenets have spread across the world. It started with the German branch of Rosicrucian's, spread to England, then came to the United states with the first settlers.

The Illuminati have 3 main branches: the Germanic branch, which oversees the others, the British branch, which handles finances, and the French/Russian branch. All 3 branches are represented in both the United States and Canada, as well as every country in the world.

HOW THE ILLUMINATI ARE ORGANIZED IN THE UNITED STATES:

The Illuminati have groups in every major city of the United States. They originally entered the U.S. through Pittsburgh, Pa., and from there, spread across the US. There are 18 cities across the US, which are considered major "power centers" for Illuminati power and/or influence. These include: Washington, DC and the surrounding areas; Albany, New York; Pittsburgh, Pa. the "golden triangle" of the Winston Salem, Raleigh, NC area, Minneapolis, Minn, Ann Arbor, Mich, Wichita, Kan., Phoenix, Az., Portland, Or., Flagstaff, Az., Seattle, Wash., Houston, TX., Los Angeles, CA. and surrounding areas, Atlanta, Ga., New Orleans, La., Springfield, Miss. Other cities are important to the Illuminati, as all, but these cities funnel money for them, conduct research, and often regional councils sit within them.

HIERARCHY OF THE ILLUMINATI

The Illuminati have organized their society along extremely hierarchical, or stratified, levels. In fact, the top levels are known as:

Hierarchical level: The Illuminati have divided the United States into 7 geographical regions; each region has its own regional council, composed of 13 members, with an advisory board of 3 elders to each one. These regions interact for purposes of finances; personnel; teaching, etc. Beneath each regional council, is a local council. This is a council of 13 members, the head of whom sits on the regional council, and gives it information about the local groups underneath his leadership. The local council will also have an advisory council of 3.

A local leadership council in a large metropolitan area might look like this:

- Head of local council (reports to regional council)
- Two intermediaries (report all activities under leader to him)
- Four administrators (oversee finances, administer, set up group activities)
- Six head trainers (over trainers in local groups, teach other trainers)

Underneath the above leadership council, will be six people designated as informers or intermediaries, who go to the local group meetings, interact with local group leaders, and report to the leadership council.

Anarchical level: the levels below the leadership council are known as the anarchical levels. Underneath the intermediate level, is the local group level. It will look like this:

Local "Sister groups" (will vary in number, according to the size of the city, or cities, in the area). A large metropolitan area may have anywhere from ten to twenty seven groups.

Each sister group will be headed up by:

A high priest and priestess: this job is rotated every 3 years, to allow different people within the group to take on leadership roles. Each group will also have different members, with specific roles/jobs within the group. These roles will be addressed in Chapter 2.

One thing that I would like to emphasize is the fact that the Illuminati today are generational. There members are born into the group, which is highly organized, as described above. The set up discussed above is representative, with minor variations, of most major metropolitan regions of the United States. Smaller population centers will be organized under similar guidelines, but will be umbrellaed together with several cities within the region to create the local leadership council.

HOW THE ILLUMINATI MAKE MONEY

The Illuminati are involved in many areas of making money, as they need continued financing to survive. There are several illegal enterprises that they are involved in, as well as legal ones.

- **Drug running:** The Illuminati linked up with the Mafia and the Columbians, years ago, to help each other out with bringing drugs into the United States. They also provide couriers for taking drugs and money out of the States. The Illuminists are generally wealthy businessmen, who have 4 layers of people underneath them. The fourth layer down actually has contact with the people in the drug industry. They never identify themselves as Illuminists; only as people interested in investing, with a guaranteed profit, and are highly secretive. In return, the local groups supply people willing to be couriers of money or drugs, or people willing to help cover for the local operations.

- **Pornography:** The Illuminati are linked in many cities with pornography/prostitution/child prostitution/ and white slavery sales. Again, several layers are present, as a buffer, between the true "management" and those either engaged in the activities, or in paying for/funding and eventually being paid for the activities.

- **Children:** are often supplied from the local cult groups, and taught to be child prostitutes (and later, adult prostitutes); are photographed and filmed in every type of pornography available, including "snuff films" and violent films.

- **Gun running:** The Illuminati and other groups are also involved in international gun sales and shipments. The Illuminists have well trained couriers who will cross international and state lines. These couriers are highly secretive, and will not reveal their sources, on pain of suicide or assassination. These people are accountable to others above them, with two more "buffer layers" of people above these, before the person in the Illuminati with money, who helps fund this, is found.

- **Buying access codes for military computers:** The Illuminati will have people from all strata of civilian life trained to go and make pickups near or on military bases. A typical person used might be the innocent looking wife of a military person, a local businessman, or even a college student. There is a contact inside the base, also a dissociative Illuminist, who brings the information to the outside contact. Occasionally, the contact person is paid with money, information, or goods. The military computer codes are changed on random schedules; the Illuminati have at least 5 or 6 contacts on each major base, who alert them when the codes are getting ready to change, on pain of death. The Illuminists like having access to military computers, because that will gain them entrance to closed files the world over.

- **Hiring and selling assassinations:** this is done worldwide, more in Europe than in the States. These people are paid big money to do either a private or political assassination. The money is paid either to the assassin, or to the trainer; usually they both divide the fee The assassin is offered protection in another country for awhile, until the trail runs cold. If the kill is done in Europe they may be sent to the far east or the U.S., and vice versa if the kill is done in the U.S. The Illuminati have a wide arena of places and false identities to hide these people, unless for some reason they want the assassin disposed of as well. Then, he/she is caught and immediately executed.

- **Mercenaries/military trainers:** guess who gets paid money to come in and train paramilitary groups? Who has training camps all over the states of Montana, Nevada, and North Dakota? Who occasionally will offer their expertise in return for a large financial reward? They never advertise themselves as Illuminati, unless the group is known to be sympathetic to their cause. Instead, these are tough, cold, brutal military trainers, who offer to teach these groups in return for money, or even better, a promise to affiliate with their group in return (loyalty in return for knowledge). More and more paramilitary groups have been brought into the Illuminati this way, without their full knowledge of who and what the group really is. This gives the Illuminists a way to monitor these groups (their trainers report on them, and their activities), and it can be useful to have trained military groups that they can call on someday.

- **Banking:** The original Illuminists were bankers, and they have highly trained financiers to organize their money, and funnel the above illicit funds into more "respectable" front groups/ organizations. They will also start benevolent charities, community organizations, etc., as fronts, and funnel the money from a broad base into these groups. The Illuminati particularly pride themselves on their money making and manipulation skills, and their ability to cover their paper trails expertly, through layer after layer.

All banking trails eventually will lead to Belgium, the Illuminati financial center for the world. These are some of the major money making enterprises that the Illuminati are engaged in. They have a lot of financial resources, backing their enterprises, which means that in reality they can engage the best lawyers, accountants, etc. to help cover their trail as well.

CHAPTER TWO

JOBS IN THE ILLUMINATI (OR WHY THEY SPEND ALL THAT TIME TRAINING PEOPLE)

To understand generational programming, it helps to understand WHY the cult goes to the amount of trouble that it does to place programming into people. Training represents time and effort, and no one- especially a cult member- will spend that amount of energy unless there will be a return on the investment. This will be a simple overview of some of the more common jobs in the cult. It is not meant to be exhaustive, or in any way considered to be complete.

The cult has a very organized hierarchy of jobs. Like any large organization, in order to run smoothly, it needs people who are well trained in their jobs- so well trained, that they can do their tasks without even thinking about them. To maintain secrecy, this group must also have people completely dedicated to not revealing their roles in the cult- even under threat of death or punishment. The cult wants members who are completely loyal to the group and its tenets, who never question the orders they are given. These qualities in group members ensure the continuance of the cult, and that its secrets are never revealed to the outside world.

Here is a sampling of some jobs in the cult (not listed in order of priority)

- **Informers:** These people are trained to observe details and conversations with photographic recall. They are trained to report to their local cult leader or hierarchy, or trainer, and will download large amounts of information under hypnotic trance. Detailed knowledge of conversations or even documents can often be retrieved in this manner. They are often used as "plants" to gather information in both governmental settings, and within the cult meetings.

- **Breeders:** These people are often chosen from childhood to have and breed children. They may be chosen according to bloodlines, or given in arranged marriages or cult alliances, to "elevate" the children. A parent will often sell the services of a child as a breeder to the local cult leader in return for favors or status. These children are rarely used as a sacrifice; usually they are given to others in the cult to adopt or raise, but the breeder is told that any child born to her was "sacrificed" to prevent her looking for the child. Occasionally, in anarchical cults, a local leader or parent will have a child as the result of an incestuous liaison. Such a child is given away or killed, but the mother will be told the child was given away to a distant branch, and must be given up.

- **Prostitutes:** Prostitutes can be a male or female of any age. They are trained from earliest childhood to give sexual favors to one or more adults in return for payment to the child's parents or their local cult group. Occasionally, the prostitute may be given to a member of the cult, on a temporary basis, as a "reward" for a job well done. Child prostitution is a big business for the cult, and training very young children in this role is taken very seriously. Child prostitutes are also used to blackmail political figures or leadership outside the cult.

- **Pornography**A child used in pornography (which may include bestiality) can also be of any age or sex. Child pornography is also big business in the cult, and includes snuff films. Children are trained in this role from preschool on, often with the help or approval of the child's parents. The parents are paid or given favors by the cult in return for selling their child or allowing their child to be trained in this area.

- **Media personnel**These are very bright, verbal people. They will be sent to journalism school and will work for local or regional media upon graduation. These individuals have many contacts within the organization as well as the outside world. They write books and articles sympathetic to the Illuministic viewpoint without ever revealing their true affiliation. They will tend to do biased research in their articles, favoring only one viewpoint, such as denying the existence of DID or ritual abuse. For instance, they will interview only psychiatrists/psychologists sympathetic to this viewpoint and will skew data to present a convincing picture to the general public. If necessary, they will outright lie or make up data to support their viewpoint. There are members of groups whose people have been purposely trained to try and help formulate public opinion on the nonexistence of the cult (i.e., cults don't exist, no rational person would believe this "mass hysteria"). The Illuminists believe that to control the media is to control the thinking of the masses. For this reason, they take training media personnel quite seriously. Helpers at rituals Cleaners clean up meticulously after rituals. They will scour the site after a ceremony, rake the area, etc. They are taught this job from preschool years on.

- **Preparers:** set up tables, cloths, candles, and paraphernalia quickly and efficiently. This job is learned from infancy on.

- **Readers:** read from the book of Illumination or local group archives; they also keep copies of sacred literature in a safe vault and are trained in ancient languages. Readers are valued for their clear speaking voices and ability to dramatize important passages and bring them to life.

- **Cutters:** are taught to dissect animal or human sacrifices (they are also known as the "slicers and dicers" of the cult). They can do a kill quickly, emotionlessly, and efficiently. They are trained from early childhood on.

- **Chanters:** sing, sway, or lead choruses of sacred songs on high holy occasions.

- **High Priest/Priestess:** The person who holds this job is changed every few years in most groups, although it may be held longer in smaller, more rural groups. These people administrate and lead their local cult group as well as coordinate jobs within the cult, give assignments, and pass on meeting dates given from the local hierarchy or leadership council. They also will activate the local group's telephone tree, evaluate their local group members for job performance, and lead in all spiritual activities. They report to the local or regional leadership council over their group.

- **Trainers:** These people teach local group members their assigned jobs and monitor the performance of these jobs at local group meetings or after an assigned task. These people report to the high priest/priestess over their group, as ell as to the local head trainer on leadership council.

- **Punishers**These are the people who brutally punish/discipline members caught breaking rules or acting outside of or above their authority. They are universally despised by other cult members, although they will be praised for a job well done by the local high priest or priestess. Usually physically strong, they will employ any method deemed necessary to prevent a recurrence of the undesired behavior. Punishment may be public or private, depending upon the severity of the infraction. Each local group has several punishers.

- **Trackers:** These people will track down and keep an eye on members who attempt to leave their local group. They are taught to use dogs, guns, taser, and all necessary tracking techniques. They are also adept at using the internet to monitor a person's activities. They will track credit card use, checks written, and employ other methods to find a missing person.

- **Teachers:** These people teach group classes to children to indoctrinate cult philosophy, languages, and specialized areas of endeavor.

- **Child care:** These people care for very young children when the adults are at local group meeting. Usually care is for young infants only. After age two, children are routinely engaged in some form of group activity led by trainers of the youngest children. Infant child care workers are usually quiet and coldly efficient.

- **Couriers:** These members run guns, money, drugs, or illegal artifacts across state or national lines. Usually they are people who are young and single without outside accountability. They are trained in the use of firearms to get out of difficult situations. They must be reliable and able to get past any anticipated barriers.

- **Commanding officers:** These people oversee military training in the local groups and help ensure the smooth running of these exercises. They will delegate jobs to those ranking under them and are responsible to the local leadership council. The council will have at least one member on it representing the military branch of the Illuminati. In addition, there are many military- related jobs beneath the commanding officers.

- **Behavioral scientists:** These individuals often oversee the training in local and regional groups. These students of human behavior are intensely involved in data collection and human experimentation in the name of the pursuit of knowledge of human behavior in the scientific realm. They are almost universally cold, methodical, impersonal people and will employ any methods to study trauma and its effects on the human personality. Their main interest centers around implementing programming and cult control in the most efficient and lasting manner.

There are many other jobs inside the cult. The cult spends quite a bit of its time getting people to do these jobs for them for FREE, which is why they PROGRAM people to believe they are doing their "family" and the world a service. The reality, of course, is that the individual is being abused and taken advantage of by the cult.

CHAPTER THREE

CONSPIRACY THEORY TWO, OR THE ILLUMINATI PLAN TO RULE THE WORLD (ALSO KNOWN AS "NOVUS ORDEM SECLORUM")

Prior to discussing actual programming techniques, it is important to understand the philosophy underlying why the Illuminists are programming people. All groups have goals, and the Illuminists are no exception. Money making is not their final goal - it is a means to an end. This end point, or goal, is no less than to rule the world. The Illuminati has a set plan similar to the Soviet Union's previous "5- year" and "10- year " plans. This is what the Illuminists themselves believe and teach their followers as gospel truth.

Whether they will actually succeed is another matter altogether. The following is the Illuminist agenda at ALL levels of the Illuminati. As with any goal, the Illuminati has specific steps which it plans to implement to reach its objectives. Briefly, each region of the United States has "nerve centers" or power bases for regional activity. The United States has been divided up into seven major geographical regions. Each region has localities within it that contain military compounds and bases that are hidden in remote, isolated areas or on large private estates.

These bases are used intermittently to teach and train generational Illuminati in military techniques, hand- to-hand combat, crowd control, use of arms, and all aspects of military warfare. Why? Because the Illuminists believe that our government, as we know it, as well as the governments of most nations around the world, are destined to collapse. These will be planned collapses, and they will occur in the following ways:

The Illuminati has planned first for a financial collapse that will make the great depression look like a picnic. This will occur through the maneuvering of the great banks and financial institutions of the world, through stock manipulation, and interest rate changes. Most people will be indebted to the federal government through bank and credit card debt, etc. The governments will recall all debts immediately, but most people will be unable to pay and will be bankrupted. This will cause generalized financial panic which will occur simultaneously worldwide, as the Illuminists firmly believe in controlling people through finances.

Next there will be a military takeover, region by region, as the government declares a state of emergency and martial law. People will have panicked, there will be an anarchical state in most localities, and the government will justify its move as being necessary to control panicked citizens. The cult trained military leaders and people under their direction will use arms as well as crowd control techniques to implement this new state of affairs. This is why so many survivors under 36 years of age report having military programming. People who are not Illuminists or who are not sympathetic to their cause, will resist. The Illuminists expect this and will be (and are BEING) trained in how to deal with this eventuality. They are training their people in hand-to- hand combat, crowd control, and, if necessary, will kill to control crowds. The Illuminati is training their people to be prepared for every possible reaction to the takeover. Many mind control victims will also be called into duty with preset command codes. These codes are meant to call out a new, completely cult loyal presenting system. Shatter codes programmed under trauma will be used to destroy or bury non-cult loyal alters.

Military bases will be set up, in each locality (actually, they are already here, but are covert). In the next few years, they will go above ground and be revealed. Each locality will have regional bases and leaders to which they are accountable. The hierarchy will closely reflect the current covert hierarchy.

About five years ago, when I left the Illuminati, approximately 1% of the US population was either part of the Illuminati, sympathetic to it, or a victim of Mind Control (and therefore considered useable).

While this may not sound like many, imagine 1% of the population highly trained in the use of armaments, crowd control, psychological and behavioral techniques, armed with weapons and linked to paramilitary groups.

These people will also be completely dedicated to their cause. The Illuminati firmly believes that it can easily overcome the other 99% of the population, most of whom are untrained, or poorly trained, such as "weekend hunters." Even the local military will be overcome as the Illuminati will have regional cell groups with highly trained leaders. They also count on the element of surprise helping them during their takeover. Many of the highest leaders in the militia branch of the Illuminati are or have been officers in the military, and so already have a good knowledge of which techniques will work best to overcome a region's or locality's defenses.

After the military takeover, the general population will be given a chance to either espouse the Illuminati's cause, or reject it (with imprisonment, pain, even death being possible punishments). These people very much believe that the intelligent, or "enlightened" or Illuminated, were born to rule. They are arrogant, and consider the general population as "dumb sheep" who will be easily led if offered strong leadership, financial help in an unstable world economy, and dire consequences if the person rebels. Their utter ruthlessness, and ability to implement this agenda, should not be minimized.

The Illuminati banking leaders, such as the Rothschilds, the Van derBilts, the Rockefellers, the Carnegies, and the Mellons, as examples, will reveal themselves, and offer to "save" the floundering world economy. A new system of monetary exchange, based on an international monetary system, and based between Cairo, Egypt, and Brussels, Belgium, will be set up. A true "one world economy", creating the longed for "one world order", will become reality.

There is more to the Illuminist agenda, but these are the basics of it. This agenda is what the Illuminati really, truly, believe, teach, and train for. They are willing to give their lives up in this cause, in order to teach the next generation, as they believe that their children are their legacy. I was told that my children's generation would see this takeover, sometime in the 21st century. At present, the Illuminati have quietly and covertly fostered their takeover plan by their goals of the infiltration of:

1. The media
2. The banking system
3. The educational system
4. The government, both local and federal
5. The sciences
6. The churches

They are currently, and have been working the last several hundred years, on taking over these 6 areas. They do NOT go to an institution, and say "hi, I'm a local Illuminist, and I'd like to take over your bank). Instead, they begin by having several people quietly invest funds over several years, gradually buying more and more shares in the bank (or other institution that they wish to control), until they have a financial controlling interest in it. They never openly disclose their agenda, or their cult activities, as often they are amnesic to them. These are well respected, "Christian" appearing business leaders in the community. The image in the community is all important to an Illuminist; they will do anything to maintain a normal, respected facade, and DESPISE exposure. On one leadership in a major metropolitan city, where I was a member, there sat: one head of the local small business administration; one CEO of a government defense firm; one principal of a Christian school; one vice mayor of the city; one journalist; one nurse; one doctor; one behavioral psychologist, one army Colonel, and one navy Commander. All except one attended church weekly; all were well respected within the community.

NONE of them appeared "evil", or "marked".

If you met them in person, you would probably instantly like any of these intelligent, verbal, likeable, even charismatic people. This is their greatest cover, since we often expect great evil to "appear" evil, led by media portrayals of evil as causing changes in the face and demeanor of people, or marking them like the biblical Cain. None of the Illuminists that I have known, had unkind, or evil appearing, persona in their daytime lives, although some were dysfunctional, such as being alcoholics. The dissociation that drives the Illuminists is their greatest cover for being undetected at this time. Many, if not most, of these people are completely unaware of the great evil that they are involved in, during the night.

There are other groups which are not actually part of the Illuminati, but the Illuminati are aware of them. The Illuminati are not the only group that follows esoteric practices, or worships ancient deities or demons. They encourage divisiveness between different groups (divide and conquer is one of their ruling principles), and are not concerned about other groups. Instead, they will often welcome them into their umbrella, if possible. This has been happening more and more in recent years, as the Illuminati trade teaching their training principles, which are considered the best by most secretive groups, in exchange for loyalty to the Illuminati. They will send their trainers to these groups, and the trainers will report to the local regional council.

In the political arena, the Illuminists will fund both sides of a race, because their greatest maxim is that "out of chaos comes order", or the discipline of anarchy. That is why they sent arms to, and funded, both sides of both the great World Wars in this century. They believe that history is a game, like chess; that only out of strategy, fighting, conflict, and testing can the strong emerge. I no longer agree with this philosophy, but at one time, I did, with all my heart. Hopefully, as these people and their agenda are exposed the common man will rise up against this intended rule to be foisted upon an unsuspecting mankind.

SVALI

CHAPTER FOUR

HOW THE ILLUMINATI PROGRAM PEOPLE: AN OVERVIEW OF SOME BASIC TYPES OF PROGRAMMING

In the first few chapters, I defined Illuminism, its reach, and some of the philosophy, money making enterprises, and agendas that help explain WHY they program people. I believe that these are important to understand, as a preface to the next few chapters. Why? The programming techniques that I will describe take an incredible amount of effort, time, dedication, and planning on the part of the cult to place in the individual. Only a very motivated group of people would spend the time it takes to do this. These chapters are very hard for me to write, as an individual, since my role in the cult was that of a programmer. So, the very techniques you will be reading about were often those that I used to place programming in individuals that I worked with. I no longer do these things, nor do I espouse doing them; the reason I am writing this book is that I believe that therapists who work with DID, as well as survivors, deserve to know WHAT is done to people, HOW it is done, as well as be given some ideas on how to undo the programming that the cult places in people.

First, I would like to address unintentional programming versus intentional programming. This is also known as the environmental milieu the child is raised in. The programming of a generational Illuminati infant often begins before its birth (this will be addressed later) but once it is born, the very environment the infant is raised in becomes a form of programming. Often, the infant is raised in a family environment that combines daytime abandonment with dysfunction in the parental figures. The infant soon learns that the nighttime, and cult activities, are the truly important ones. The infant may be deprived of attention, or even abused, in the daytime; and is only treated as special, or "seen" by the parent, in the cult setting. This can lead to very young alters around the core or core splits, who feel "invisible", abandoned, rejected, unworthy of love or attention, or that they don't even exist, unless they are doing a job for their "family".

Another milieu and conditioning process the infant must face is that the adults around him/her are INCONSISTENT, since the adults in a generational cult family are almost always also multiple, or DID. This sets up a reality for the infant/toddler that the parents act one way at home; an entirely different way at cult gatherings; and yet a different way in normal society.

Since these are the infant's earliest experiences of adults and adult behaviors, it has no choice but to accept this reality that human beings act in shockingly different ways in different settings. While unintentional, this sets the infant up for later dissociation, in mimicry of the adults around it.

INTENTIONAL PROGRAMMING

Intentional programming of an infant in the Illuminati often begins before birth. Prenatal splitting is well known in the cult, as the fetus is very capable of fragmenting in the womb due to trauma. This is usually done between the seventh and ninth month of pregnancy. Techniques used include: placing headphones on the mother's abdomen, and playing loud, discordant music (such as some modern classical pieces, or even Wagner's operas). Loud, heavy rock has also been used. Other methods include having the mother ingest quantities of bitter substances, to make the amniotic fluid bitter, or yelling at the fetus inside the womb. The mother's abdomen may be hit as well. Mild shock to the abdomen may be applied, especially when term is near, and may be used to cause premature labor, or ensure that the infant is born on a ceremonial holiday. Certain labor inducing drugs may be also given if a certain birth date is desired.

Once the infant is born, testing is begun at a very early age, usually during the first few weeks of life. The trainers, who are taught to look for certain qualities in the infant, will place it on a velvet cloth on a table, and check its reflexes to different stimuli. The infant's strength, how it reacts to heat, cold, and pain are all tested. Different infants react differently, and the trainers are looking for dissociative ability, quick reflexes, and reaction times. They are also encouraging early dissociation in the infant with these tests.

The infant will also be abused, to create fragments. Methods of abuse can include: rectal probes; digital anal rape; electric shocks at low levels to the fingers, toes, and genitalia; cutting the genitalia in ritual circumstances (in older infants). The intent is to begin fragmentation before a true ego state develops, and customize the infant to pain and reflexive dissociation from pain (yes, even tiny infants dissociate; I have seen it time and time again; they will glow blank and limp, or glassy, in the face of continued trauma.)

Isolation and abandonment programming will sometimes be begun as well, in a rudimentary sense. The infant is abandoned, or uncared for by adults, intentionally during the daytime, then picked up, soothed, cleaned up and paid attention to in the context of preparing for a ritual or group gathering. This is done in order to help the infant associate night gatherings with "love" and attention, and to help the bonding process to the cult, or "family". The infant will be taught to associate maternal attention with going to rituals, and eventually will associate cult gatherings with feelings of security.

As the infant grows older, i.e. at 15 to 18 months, more fragmenting is intentionally done by having the parents as well as cult members abuse the infant more methodically. This is done by intermittently soothing, bonding with the infant, then shocking it on its digits; the infant may be dropped from heights to a mat or mattress and laughed at as it lays there startled and terrified, crying. It may be placed in cages for periods of time, or exposed to short periods of isolation. Deprivation of food, water, and basic needs may begin later in this stage. All of these methods are done in order to create intentional dissociation in the infant. The infant of this age may be taken to group meetings, but outside of special occasions, or dedications, will have no active role yet in the cult setting. The small infants are usually left with a cult member, or caretaker, who watches them during the group's activities; this caretaker role is usually rotated among lower level or teenage members.

Between the ages of 20 and 24 months, the toddler may begin the "steps of discipline" which the Illuminati use to teach their children. The age the child begins them will vary, depending upon the group, the parent, the trainer, and the child. These "steps of discipline" would be better called "steps of torment and abuse" as their purpose is to create a highly dissociative child, out of touch with their feelings, who is completely and unthinkingly loyal to the cult. The order of the steps may also be varied a little, depending on the whims of the trainer or parents.

I will first discuss the first five steps of discipline: (note: these steps may vary somewhat from region to region, but most follow this outline at least roughly, even if not in the same order)

FIRST STEP: TO NOT NEED

The small toddler/child is placed in a room without any sensory stimulus, usually a training room with gray, white, or beige walls. The adult leaves and the child is left alone, for periods of time: these may vary from hours, to an entire day as the child grows older. If the child begs the adult to stay, and not leave, or screams, the child is beaten, and told that the periods of isolation will increase until they learn to stop being weak. The ostensible purpose of this discipline is to teach the child to rely on its own internal resources, and not on outside people ("strengthen it"). What it actually does is create a huge terror of abandonment within the child. When the adult, or trainer, returns to the room, the child is often found rocking itself, or hugging itself in a corner, occasionally almost catatonic from fear. The trainer will then "rescue" the child, feed and give it something to drink and bond with the child as their "savior". The trainer will tell them the "family" told the trainer to rescue the child, because its family "loves" it.

The trainer will instill cult teachings, at this point, into the helpless, fearful, and almost insanely grateful child who has just been "rescued" from isolation. The trainer will reinforce in the child over and over how much it "needs " its family, who just rescued it from death by starvation or abandonment. This will teach the very young toddler to associate comfort and security with bonding with its trainer, who may be one of its parents, and being with "family" members. The cult is very aware of child developmental principles, and has developed exercises like the above after hundreds of years of teaching very young children.

SECOND STEP: TO NOT WANT

This step is very similar to the first step, and actually reinforces it. It will be done intermittently with the first step over the next few years of the child's life. Again, the child is left alone in a training room, or isolated room, without food or water for a long period of time. An adult will enter the room, with a large pitcher of ice water, or food. If the child asks for either, as the adult is eating or drinking in front of the child, he/she is severely punished for being weak and needy. This step is reinforced, until the child learns not to ask for food or water unless it is offered first. The ostensible reason the cult gives for this step is that it creates a child who is strong, and can go without food and water for longer and longer periods of time. The real reason this is done is that it creates a child who is completely dissociated from its own needs for food, water, or other comforts, who becomes afraid to ask outside adults for help. This creates in the child a hyper-vigilance as she/he learns to look for outside adults for cues on when it is okay to fulfill needs, and not to trust her/his own body signals. The child is already learning to look outside itself to others to learn how it should think or feel, instead of trusting its own feelings. The cult now becomes the locus of control for the child.

THIRD STEP: TO NOT WISH

The child is placed in a room with favorite toys, or objects. A kind adult comes into the room and engages the child in play. This adult my be a friend, aunt, parent, or trainer. The child and adult may engage in fantasy play about the child's secret wishes, dreams, or wants. This will occur on several occasions, and the child's trust is slowly gained. At some later point, the child is severely punished for any aspect of wishing or fantasy shared with the adult, including the destruction of favorite toys, going in and undoing or destroying secret safe places the child may have created, or even destroying non cult protectors. This step is repeated, with variations, many times over the ensuing years. Occasionally, the child's siblings, parents, or friends will be used to reveal inside fantasies the child has revealed to them during the daytime, or in unguarded moments. The ostensible reason the cult gives for this step is to create a child who doesn't fantasize, who is more outwardly directed, less inwardly directed. In other words, the child is to look to adults for permission in all aspects of its life, including internal. The reality is that this step destroys all safe places the child has created internally, to retreat from the horrors it is experiencing. This step creates in the child the feeling that there is no true safety, that the cult will find out everything it thinks. Exercises like this are also used to create young alters in the child who will self report to the cult trainers any secret safe places, or covert wishes against the cult, that other alters have. This will then begin to set up intersystem hostility and divisiveness, which the cult will manipulate throughout the person's life span in order to control them.

FOURTH STEP: THE SURVIVAL OF THE FITTEST

This step is used in order to begin creating perpetrator alters in the young child. ALL CULT MEMBERS WILL BE EXPECTED TO BECOME PERPETRATORS; THIS BEGINS IN EARLY CHILDHOOD.

The child is brought into a room where there is a trainer and another child of approximately the same age, or slightly younger, that the child being taught. The child is severely beaten, for a long period of time, by the trainer, then told to hit the other child in the room, or they will be beaten further. If the child refuses, it is punished severely, the other child is punished as well, then the child is told to punish the other child. If the child continues to refuse, or cries, or tries to hit the trainer instead, they will continue to be beaten severely, and told to hit the other child, to direct its anger at the other child. This step is repeated until the child finally complies. This step is begun around age 2 to 2 1/2, and is used to create aggressive perpetrator alters in the young child. As the child becomes older, the punishing tasks become more and more brutal. Children are expected to become perpetrators of others at very young ages, and will "practice" on children younger than themselves, with the encouragement and rewarding by the adults around them. They will also be mimicking these adults, who role model perpetration constantly as normal. The child will be taught that this is the acceptable outlet for the aggressive impulses and rage that are created by the brutality the child is constantly being exposed to.

FIFTH STEP: THE CODE OF SILENCE

Many, many different stratagems are used to put this in, starting at around the age of two years old, when a child starts becoming more verbal. Usually, after a ritual or group gathering, the child is asked about what they saw, or heard, during the meeting. Like most obedient young children, they will comply. They are immediately severely beaten, or tortured, and a new alter is created, who is told to keep or guard the memories of what was seen, on pain of their life. The new part always agrees. The child and this new part are put through a ceremony of swearing to never ever tell; and alters are created whose job it is to kill the body, if the other parts ever remember.

The child is also put through severe psychological torture to ensure that it will never be tempted to tell, including: being buried alive; near drowning; watching "traitor's deaths" involving slow painful torture, such as being burned, or skinned alive; being buried with a partially rotted corpse and being told that they will become a corpse like it if they ever tell, etc. The scenarios go on and on, invented by people with endlessly cruel imaginations, in order to ensure the secrecy of the young child. These methods have been perfected over hundreds of years of practice by the cult with its children. The reason these things are done is self evident: the cult is involved in criminal activities, as explained in the first few chapters of this book, and they want to ensure the continued silence of its children. This is one reason why the cult has survived so long, and with its continued shroud of secrecy; why more survivors are afraid/ unwilling to disclose their abuse. In order to reveal cult secrets, a child must go against some of the most tremendously horrendous psychological trauma and abuse imaginable; even as an adult, the survivor has difficulty putting these things aside, when discussing their abuse. Children and adults alike are told that if they ever tell, they will be hunted down and shot (the assassin training lets the child know that this is no idle threat); that they will be tortured slowly. The child will be exposed to setups and role plays throughout their growing up that reinforces this step.

SUGGESTIONS THAT MAY HELP

I believe in also offering some ideas on how to undo some of the above mentioned programming, as I do not believe in knowledge, only for knowledge's sake. The survivor often needs tools, in order to try and undo some of the horrendous abuse that the cult places him/her through, especially as memories of these things occur. THESE ARE JUST

MEANT AS HELPFUL HINTS AND DO NOT REPLACE THE ADVICE OF A GOOD THERAPIST.

1. **Early milieu programming:**

This is difficult to undo, since it hits on core abandonment issues, and rejection, for the survivor. This will often have been the survivor's very first, earliest experiences as an infant, involving its relationship with its parents and primary family members. Working on this requires the whole hearted effort of all alter systems inside, to join in nurturing the core splits who experienced severe parental rejection, and the cognitive recognition that the DAYTIME was important, too; that the adults around the infant were the unhealthy ones. The infant's often feel unlovable, overly needy, depressed; but nurturing alters inside can help comfort them, and share the reality that the infant really was loveable, no matter what the outside adults around it were like. Here, too, an outside supportive therapist, and a strong, nurturing faith system, can help tremendously in the healing process, as new messages are brought in to the abandoned, wounded parts. Sorting through what happened, grieving over the real issues of abandonment, and bringing reality to very young, deeply wounded parts will take time.

2. **Early intentional fragmentation: (ages 0 to 24 months)**

Usually there are cognitive parts of the survivor inside, who have never ever forgotten the abuse, and can help share the cognitive reality of the abuse with the amnesic alters. This should be done extremely slowly, since this first abuse was done quite early in life. Creating an internal nursery, with safe toys, objects, can help. Older nurturing adult alters inside can help hold and care for the wounded infants inside the nursery, while acknowledging and grieving over the abuse which occurred. It is important to believe an validate the young parts when they come forward to share. Allowing them nonverbal ways of expressing themselves can help, as these are quite young parts, who often cannot talk yet. Having older children inside who are close to the infants verbalize their wants, needs, and fears can also help, as often the youngest parts inside do not trust ANY adults, even internal ones. A strong ,caring outside therapist is also important to healing, by modeling healthy nurturing to a system that may have no concept of this, while balancing the need of the infant for outside nurture with the need for the internal system(s) to learn their own self nurture techniques. Internal helpers can reach the infants, ground them, share present reality (that the body is older, the infants are safe, etc. These helpers may be internal older children, as mentioned before). The survivor may also want to find support adults when possible, who can help with modeling healthy caring with good boundaries.

A THERAPIST OR FRIEND CANNOT RE-PARENT THE SURVIVOR. The survivor will long for this, but realistically, the survivor has one set of parents, good or bad, or sadly, even terrible. No outside person can come in and redo the complete re-parenting of another. What the therapist and support person can offer will be caring, empathy, listening, while the survivor grieves over the loss of adequate nurture. They can offer friendship or empathy with good boundaries. They cannot become the survivor's parents, or therapy will not progress. Instead, enmeshment will begin.

3. The First Five Steps of Discipline (there are twelve total; others will be addressed in later chapters)

Try to find the parts that experienced the abuse. This may mean doing system mapping (drawing pictures of what things look like inside), and going to the cognitives (intellectuals) or controllers (head honchos inside) for information. An internal helper, or recorder, may also be extremely helpful in doing this.

Allow these parts to slowly acknowledge the agony that they experienced during their deprivation: heat (being held over a fire, or stove); cold (such as being placed in freezers, or ice, for example), lack of food, etc. Encourage the sharing of the cognitive portion of the memories first, while allowing amnesic alters to grieve over "hearing about" these things. Allow them time to absorb hearing about these traumas, as they occurred over several years during early childhood, and will take time to assimilate.

Healing can't be rushed. Allow feeling alters later to step forward, and share their feelings, while more cognitive or helper parts are inside holding their hands, grounding them to the here and now throughout the process of remembering Be prepared for floods of emotion at times, as well as body memories, as the abuse is recalled. A group of inside people can be designated as a "grounding team" to help ground these parts as they step forward and share their memories.

Remembering safely assumes that the person has a qualified therapist, and also has laid the groundwork for good intrasystem cooperation, as discussed above. Memory work should not be done until there is good communication and cooperation inside, or the person will be overwhelmed by the memories as they come out. They will be flooded and re-traumatized instead of helped, and may de-compensate.

With good communication, memories can be brought out a little at a time, in manageable pieces, while cognitive alters continually help keep the survivor from going completely into the memory, and they can also help ground the more wounded parts.

The cult will put people through certain types of programming in order to achieve a specific goal: separating the intellect, or cognition, form the feelings in a person. Cognitive alters in these systems are always considered "higher" than the feeling alters; cognitive alters are taught to "pass down" their feelings to the "lower" feeling alters. While these labels are untrue, the cognitive alters will fear feeling the intense, overwhelming emotions that caused them to split further and further from the more limbic, or feeling alters internally. This will drive continued system divisiveness in the survivor. It is important that cognitive parts realize that the feeling alters are part of them; that they can practice sharing their feelings in SMALL steps without needing to be flooded, or overwhelmed.

A reminder: EXTERNAL SAFETY IS PARAMOUNT TO UNDOING INSIDE PROGRAMMING.

You HAVE to be able to promise these parts external safety, and deliver on this promise, or they will understandably balk at working inside on undoing programming. Why should they try and change, only to go back and be punished again? No system will undo its own protective dissociation, if the abuse is ongoing, or it will continue to destabilize and re-dissociate over and over. This is because dismantling the dissociation would mean dismantling its own survival and protection. Stopping contact with perpetrators and having a safe therapist are the very first steps to take, before attempting to undo internal programming. A system can still work on stopping cult contact, and begin healing, while being accessed, but it will slow therapy down tremendously as the internal energy will be diverted to staying safe rather than undoing trauma. A person can heal, and most survivors are still in cult contact when they enter therapy. BUT the progress will go much more quickly once cult contact is broken. (see chapter on preventing accessing of the survivor)

CHAPTER FIVE

COLORS, METALS AND JEWEL PROGRAMMING

One form of programming that is quite common in the Illuminati is color programming. Why is it done? The answer is that trainers are human, and also quite lazy. Color programming is a simple way to organize systems, and allows the trainer to call up alters easily within a system. With the thousands of fragments that many multiples in the cult have, colors is a way of organizing them into an easily accessible group.

Also, young children recognize colors before they can read, so this training can occur quite early. It is begun at about age two in most children.

How it is done: The child is taken into a room with either white, beige, or colored walls. If the room is a neutral color, the lights in the room will be changed, so they color the room with the light's color. If "blue" is the color being imprinted, or put in, the trainer will call up a young child alter, either a controller or core split for a system. They will tell the child that they will learn how to become blue, and what blue means. The room will be bathed in blue light, as mentioned, or has been painted blue for use in this kind of programming. The trainer will be dressed in blue clothing, and may even have a blue mask on. Blue objects will be placed around the room. The alter inside the child is called up, drugged, hypnotized, and traumatized on the table. As they are awakening from the trauma, still in trance, they are told that blue is good, and that they are blue. That blue is important. That blue will protect them from harm. That blue people don't get hurt. This will go on for awhile.

They then ask the child if they want to be "blue", like the trainers. If the child says yes, they will continue on. If the child says no, it will be re-traumatized until it says yes. The child is often naked, and told it cannot wear clothing until it "earns" the right to wear beautiful blue clothing. Over and over the "safety of being blue" (ie freedom from harm) and danger of not having a color is emphasized. The children really want to be blue after a while of going through this. They may be given blue candy as a reward for choosing to become the color. They may be given blue sunglasses or tinted lenses to wear.

They are allowed to wear blue robes once they identify with the color chosen for them.

Once the child completely identifies with the color (or rather, the main alter or template for the system accepts this color), then they are taught in progressive stages, over many training sessions, what the color blue means. They are in set ups, or dramas with other blue children, where they act out the role of a "blue". They are drugged, hypnotized, traumatized, while the meaning of blue is ground in over and over. They are forced to act in "blue" ways. Different trainers and regions will assign different meanings to different colors. Many military systems are coded blue, or protective. The military alters all are called up periodically to reinforce blue training. If the trainer at a later date wants to access a blue system, they may call them up by color, or wear a piece of clothing or a scarf in the color they want to reach.

This becomes an unconscious trigger for this color to come forward. Color coding is one of the first methods that is inlayed over systems. An entire system may be color coded one color; or two or more colors may be coded in , with each system controller (most systems have three) being given a different color over its part of the system.

METALS PROGRAMMING:

Metals programming is a type of programming that many Illuminati children are given. Because it is so similar to jewels programming, I will discuss how it is done under jewels. Metals can be from bronze (lowest) to platinum (highest).

JEWELS PROGRAMMING:

Many Illuminati children will go through either metals or jewels programming, and occasionally will go through both. Jewels is considered higher than metals, and more difficult to obtain. Which is put in and when, is dependent on the child's status, its parents status, the region it is born in, the group it is born into, and the trainers that work with it.

Basically, either metals or jewels is a form of reward based programming. Here is how it works:

The child is shown a piece of jewelry such as a ring, or else a large example of the jewel (or metal) being put in. They are asked: "isn't this Amethyst, or Ruby, Emerald, Diamond) beautiful?" The child will be eager to look at it, touch it, and is encouraged to by a trainer with a soft kind voice. The trainer will ask the child, "wouldn't you like to be beautiful, like this jewel? (or metal jewelry)". The child is usually eager to be. Here is a sparkling gemstone, placed in their small hands (the training often begins between age two and three). Of course they want to be beautiful, sparkly, valued. The trainer will extol the beauty of the gem (or metal), will tell the child how special, valued, wanted gems are, and basically build up the idea of becoming like a jewel.

The child is then told that in order to become a jewel, they must "earn the right". This involves:

a.) passing through steps of discipline (see chapter three)

b.) passing "special tests"

c.) being rewarded for special achievement

Becoming a jewel (or precious metal) is dangled before the small child, like a carrot, as the reward for doing well in training sessions. The earning of one is linked to going through the rungs of the long, arduous training process expected of Illuminati children; having a jewel or metal involves stepping up in status and being praised. But the price is enduring hours of abuse called "training" but in reality is organized, systemic abuse to make the child do what the trainer wants them to become.

Over time, with the help of drugs, hypnosis, shock, and other trauma, as the child goes through it's training process, it will begin earning its jewels and/or metals, one by one. These will become full alters inside.

Amethyst is usually the first one earned, and is linked to keeping secrets, never telling, and passing the first step of discipline. Each step is linked to receiving either a jewel or precious metal.

Ruby will often be next, and is linked to sexual abuse and sexual alters inside. As the child is repeatedly sexually traumatized and survives, or creates sexual alters to please adults, they are "rewarded" by being allowed to become a ruby.

Emerald will often come later (ages 12 to 15). This is considered very precious, and is linked to family loyalty, witchcraft, and spiritual achievement. Emeralds will often have a black cat, or "familiar" linked to them.

Diamond is the highest gemstone, and not all children will earn it. It is considered a high achievement. and may not be earned until adulthood, after passing rigorous tasks. It will be the controlling alter in a gemstone system. A diamond has passed all twelve steps of discipline, plus passed unusual tests and will have highest family loyalty.

"Family jewels" are often passed down internally during training sessions with trainers and family members. All high Illuminati families will have jewels hidden in secret vaults (real, outside jewels) which have been passed down for generations.

The children will often be given jewelry to wear in the daytime, as a reminder or reward, once they pass their programming. A child may be given a ruby ring or garnet pin to wear; in fact, a grandparent or parent may insist the child wear it. On ritual occasions, the child will be allowed to wear jewelry from the family's vault, once they reach a certain status. They may be allowed to wear a ruby pendant or emerald bracelet during high rituals, and will be quite proud of the fact, since the cult is first, foremost and always an extremely status conscious group. The children pick up on this, and the adults will make a big fuss over the children who have earned the right to wear jewels. This gives them a huge incentive to earn them.

Suggestions that may help with these forms of programming :

Color programming: it is important to have good internal communication with both internal alters and an outside therapist while working on color programming. If an individual finds that certain parts believe that they are a certain color, or if this comes up in therapy, they will want to find out if possible how they came to have this belief system. Slowly discovering how the colors were put in will help. Grieving for the vast amount of deception, the amount of abuse heaped on the child, and the very young alters who were the original templates may occur. These parts may be barely verbal, and may want to draw their experiences, or use colors in collages (with the help of older parts inside), to describe to a safe outside person what their reality has been. Validating to them that they are NOT just a color, that they are part of a whole person, may help. The survivor may see colored overlays for awhile, as they are undoing this programming, as parts inside share their memories. This is normal, although it may feel uncomfortable to see objects as yellow or green, for example. Grounding oneself, having cognitives do reality orientation, and patience will help the survivor work through this time.

Jewel programming and metals may be more complex, since the child's sense of special ness, pride and status may be bound up in these alters. Rubies, emeralds and diamonds are considered "high alters" inside and are used to leadership roles, both internally and externally. Acknowledging their importance to the system; listening to them grieve at leaving the cult, which meant giving up their status externally, and giving them new positions inside that are important can help. They can become system leaders in helping the person stay safe, once they make the decision to leave the cult, and become strong allies. But they will often be among the most resistant, and even hostile, to the idea of leaving the cult at first, since they have only known and remembered being rewarded for jobs well done, and have learned to "pass down" the traumas to "lower parts" inside. They will often honestly not believe they have been abused, and will only remember being petted or allowed to lead, or being told they were special, valued.

Listening to how they feel; acknowledging that leaving means giving up things that were important to them, finding out what needs motivated them, and trying to find healthy outlets for them to get their needs met outside of cult meetings will help. Letting a jewel have leadership within, or chair internal meetings may make up for loss of external leadership when the survivor leaves the cult.

Acknowledging their importance to the survivor is also important. Recognize that these parts are EXTREMELY dissociated from their own abuse/trauma, and are in no hurry to remember. But both the survivor and a good therapist can bring reality gently to them, as they let them know that they were abused; that they are actually part of the "lower emotional parts" who were abused, and will eventually need to acknowledge this. This task takes time and good outside support to accomplish. Allow them to vent their feelings. They will often be highly cognitive at first, but feelings will come, especially grieving, then pain at having been deceived by the cult, then the anguish of realizing that the abuse they passed down to others inside was actually happening to them. They may become quite depressed at this stage, but will also lend tremendous stability and strength to the system, in staying safe and cult free, once they have reached this stage.

These are some thoughts on color, metals, and jewel programming. Other types of programming will be addressed in the next chapter.

CHAPTER SIX

BRAIN WAVE PROGRAMMING

In this chapter I will address brain wave programming. Brain wave programming, like any other programming, will depend on several factors.

These include: the child's ability to dissociate; the region of the country or which country the child grows up in; the level of ability of the trainers the child has contact with; physical resources and equipment available. There is no one "recipe" that fits every person and it would be ridiculous to state that all people who go through brain wave programming have it done the same way. More and more, programmers are talking, sharing knowledge over the net, both nationally and internationally, and sharing both successes and failures. But there is no one standardized methodology for brain wave programming. It will often be influenced by the child herself, as well as the trainer's whims. Different groups may organize the systems differently, or try to achieve different effects.

All of this said, what is brain wave programming? Simply put, brain wave programming involves having a young child go into a deep trance state, where they then learn to dissociate into a certain brain wave pattern. This is a complex skill, and not all children can achieve this. The goal is for the child to reach, for example, a consistent delta state, where delta brain waves show up on the EEG, which is attached to the child's head by electrodes in the scalp. Usually, two or even three trainers will work on one child during the initial stages. One will "prep" the child, using a hypnotic drug to induce a trance state. They will have also placed the electrodes on the head, using an abbreviated version of the method used in traditional hospital setting. If delta state is being induced, only the electrodes needed to pick up delta waves will be placed, for example. This is to save time.

The prepped child will be on a "trainer's table", and will be quite relaxed. The average child is about eight years old when this is begun, since the cerebral cortex and neurological development are not advanced enough at earlier ages (It has been tried at earlier ages, quite unsuccessfully, in the past; this practice was dropped because of the neurological damage and "failure to take rate" that trainers were seeing). The non prepping trainer will then let the child know exactly what he/she expects: that they will achieve a special state, called "delta state". The trainer tells the child, while they are in trance state, that they will know when they reach it, by the readings from the electrodes.

The trainer will tell the child alter, who has been called up to be a "template", or building block for the new system, that delta is good. They will emphasize this over and over. The child will then be shocked to increase its receptivity to learning. This also arouses the child from its drugged state and it will be more alert. It will want to please the trainer. The trainer will tell the child that she/he wants it to perform certain mental exercises. It will then give it backwards counting exercises, used to help the child achieve deeper trance states. Other verbal cues to trance down may be given. When the prepping or technical trainer sees delta waveforms, he or she will signal the verbal trainer with a hand motion. The verbal, or teaching trainer will immediately reward the child, saying, "good, you are in delta now." The trainer will caress the child, tell it what a good job it is doing. If the child bounces out of delta state, the verbal trainer will immediately become harsh, and will shock the child as punishment. The child is told that it left delta (which is "good") and needs to go back in.

The induction, counting, will be repeated until delta state is seen again, when the child is repeatedly rewarded for entering, then staying in this state for longer and longer periods. The trainers are using biofeedback principles to teach the child to consistently cue into a brainwave pattern. When the template can stay in delta pattern consistently, the template will be rewarded. This will occur over several months.

The trainers will now have a template that stays always in delta state, that they can begin splitting and using as the basis of forming a new system inside. They will do this using the tools of drugs, hypnosis and trauma. The new system created will record delta waves on an EEG if done correctly. The new system will be taught what delta means. The trainers will often flash a cue, or delta (triangle) symbol on a projector overhead, and "grind in" the delta imprinting. They will wear robes with delta signs on them, and cloth the subject in clothing or robes imprinted with the delta sign. They will teach the alters under hypnosis what deltas do, how they act. They will reward them when they comply, and shock or otherwise traumatize them if they do not act like "deltas". They will be given delta jobs. They will watch high frequency films, that show delta functions. They may build in a computer like structure to hold the system, showing pictures of its organization while the subject is under deep trance, after creating a clean slate through trauma.

These are some examples of how delta programming may be induced.

Other brain wave states will be induced in similar manners. They will often be formed from templates which are extremely young internal child alters who may be splits from core splits, as the basis for the programming. Common brain wave states used are:

Alpha: this is the most easily reached brain wave state, and also includes both the youngest and most easily accessed alters in the entire system. Young children have long periods of alpha activity and must be trained to enter other brain wave states for long periods. System access programming; access codes and sexual alters will often be placed in alpha, which may also be coded red in some systems.

Beta: this is the next most easily reached state, and is often associated with aggressive impulses. Beta state will often hold cult protectors, internal warriors, and military systems. They may be color coded blue.

Gamma: this will often hold extremely cult loyal alters, and holds more emotion than the other states, except for alpha. Suicide programming will often be layered into this system, as these alters would rather die than leave their "family". Scholarship programming may be held by this system, since they easily memorize by rote. Several languages may be spoken by different alters in this system, as the Illuminati like to program in plural linguality, with up to eight languages, both modern and ancient being spoken.

Delta: this is one of the more cognitive brain wave states, and will often be highly dissociated. It may also be the "ruling" or controlling state over the other brain wave systems. Often, delta state may be configured inside as a computer, and the delta alters will have emotionless, flat alters with photographic memories. They may hold most of the cognitive memories for the other systems, especially if extensive amnesia programming has been done. Delta state may have up to three levels of training: delta 1, delta 2, and delta 3 which will also correlate to security access allowed within the cult; i.e. access to highly confidential information. Behavioral sciences programming may be held by this system. Internal programmers, self destruct, psychotic, and shatter programming as well as other punishment programming sequences to prevent outside access or internal access to the systems may be held within delta systems. It may be color coded both orange/blue/purple, and will also often be the entry way to higher systems such as jewels or internal councils, inside.

Epsilon: this is often a "hidden system" and may hold CIA programming and high level governmental programming . Assassin programming may be held in this system, or in the beta system, depending on the trainer. Covert operations, courier operations, learning to tail a subject, or "drop a tag", disguises, getting out of difficult situations, may be handled by this system, which sees itself as chameleon-like. It may be color coded brown.

Phi/Theta/Omega programming: this represents negative spiritual programming. These are the "dark" ritual alters, who participate in blood rituals, sacrifices, and ceremonies. Internal witches, warlocks, seers, psychics, readers, and occult practitioners will be placed in this system, which has highly developed right brain and deep trance abilities. They will often be color coded black.

This is an overview of some of the more common brain wave systems. It is often placed in over a matter of years, from ages 8 to 21 being the primary ones, with occasional reinforcement of the programming from time to time.

SUGGESTIONS:

Brain wave programming is a very complex form of programming which creates automatic amnesia and communication barriers between the different brain wave states. This will also be reinforced by shock and punishment to prevent its "degradation", or undoing. Internal system controllers and programmers will also work to reinforce the programming, especially at night, when the person is asleep (physically).

All brain wave systems will have system controllers, usually set up in a group of three (the Illuminati love triads, as being the "mystical" and most stable number. They believe that systems built upon triads are extremely strong, unbreakable, and will often program in threes: three back ups, three system controllers, etc.) With the help of a good therapist, the survivor needs to get to know the internal system controllers and communicators. They are there, they have to be, because the trainers placed them there to communicate with and be accountable to them externally, and will often have complete knowledge of their own system. They will also be quite flat, and dissociated from the knowledge of their own pain or the abuse that created them. This is a distancing mechanism, and the person's survival depended on the ability of their controller to do this at one time. They will often be quite hostile, and very unwilling to look at their own abuse; they will become indignant at the idea, and claim that they are cognitive, and "above" being abused (another lie they were told by their abusers).

Time, patience, and finding out what their needs are; listening to them vent their frustration; pointing out reality (ie, the controllers, and all parts are related to each other; are part of the same person; and ALL were abused even though they were able to dissociate from their pain), and trying to help them meet their needs for recognition, acceptance, and approval will begin to allow them to question their previous loyalty. These systems are often driven by fear: fear of punishment; fear of remembering (they were often the most tortured systems in the survivor, and were promised amnesia in return for continued cooperation). Their fears are real, and should be listened to and respected, as shatter programming and flood programming are real threats to the survivor, and can cause functionality to go down.

Flood programming is a sequence put in place to punish a system if its internal programming is allowed to degrade or access to an unauthorized person, either internally or externally, is allowed. It will involve the fragments who hold highly traumatic memories, both emotional and physical, being pushed to the front where the person is "flooded" with wave after wave of memories. If this is triggered, and it frequently is if the survivor is in therapy, the first priority should be slowing the memories down. This may mean trying to reason with internal controllers or deltas who are allowing the flooding; they need to know that if the front, or previously amnesic alters down, or are re-shattered due to traumatization, it will weaken all the systems.

Bargain with them. Prayer will help in this situation. Physical safety, including inpatient therapy, may be needed if flooding or shatter programming are activated. Suicide programming is often layered in with both types, and external physical safety will be paramount for the survivor, with lots of outside accountability as they undo these intense programming sequences. Frequent reality orientation; explaining new, better jobs can help. Undoing brain wave programming should ideally only be done with lots of safe external support, which may include extra therapy sessions; hospitalization if programming that could cause loss of functionality or suicide are triggered; and should be geared towards increasing internal communication and cooperation. Alters jobs can be changed, from internal programmers to internal Deprogrammers; internal shatterers or punishers to internal protectors; internal reporters who report back to the cult can instead be asked to report internally on what the body is doing, and to keep it safe.

These are examples of possible changes. Make friends with system controllers, as they can become strong helpers and will work with the therapist to keep things safe for the survivor.

CHAPTER SEVEN

MILITARY PROGRAMMING

I want to devote an entire chapter to military programming, and how it is done. Why? As noted in chapter three, the Illuminati are emphasizing the importance of military training more and more, as part of their plan for eventual takeover. All children in the current generation are undergoing some form of military training as part of this plan.

Military training is begun quite young. It is often started by three years of age with simple exercises. The children are taken by their parents to a training area, which may be a large inside auditorium, or a remote area outside where training maneuvers are done. Tents are set up, with command centers for the different commanding officers and military trainers.

The children are taught to march in time, keeping a straight line. They are punished by being kicked, shocked with a cattle prod, or beaten with a baton if they move out of place. They will be dressed in small uniforms in imitation of the adults.

The adults will have ranks, badges and insignia indicating their level of achievement in the cult hierarchy and military. Badges and medals are given out to indicate the person's level of training and tests passed. Commanding officers are often brutal and will teach even the youngest children with harsh measures.

The children will be forced to march long distances, which increase as they get older, in any weather. They are forced to learn to cross obstacles. They will be given "fake" guns, with blanks, when they are young. These guns are perfect replicas of real guns, but fire blanks. The children are taught to load and fire all manner of firearms, both real and fake, under close adult supervision. They will spend hours learning to aim, sight, and fire these guns at targets. At first the targets are bulls eyes, but as the children get older the targets will be similar to police cut outs of humans. The children are taught to aim for the head or the heart. Later, they will graduate to realistic manikins. This is conditioning them to kill a human being.

They will be shown violent films of warfare, much more explicit and graphic than normal movies in group classes. Killing techniques will be shown in slow motion. The motif "kill or be killed" will be ground in over and over. The trainer will ask the children what mistakes the people who were killed made. Being killed is considered weakness; being a killer is considered strength.

The children will be forced, by age seven or eight, to crawl on their bellies with simulated blanks firing overhead. They are not told these are blanks and they are extremely painful if the child is hit in the back or buttocks. They quickly learn to keep down under fire. Battle conditions will be simulated as the children go through years of "boot camp" training.

They will be rewarded with merit badges for doing well, such as completing an obstacle course, or staying cool under fire. In other words, the cult creates a microcosm of real military training for their children and youth. Nazi concentration camps will be simulated, with guards and prisoners. The "guards" are usually older children or youth who have done well. The "prisoners" are younger children or those being punished for not performing well in maneuvers. There is intense pressure to want the guard role and not be a prisoner, since prisoners are locked up, beaten, kicked, and laughed at.

Hunting and tracking games where the prisoners are given a half hour lead are frequent. These may also involve the use of specially trained dogs taught to knock the quarry down but not kill them. Older children are taught to handle the dogs, and use them. Youth are taught to help the adults train the dogs.

Teens may be rewarded by becoming "youth leaders" who are allowed to plan the weeks activities. The military training will closely follow the principles of Nazi military and S.S. training. The trainers often speak in German to the children, who must learn the language. All C.O.s and high ranking adults speak in German during these exercises. They may also speak in French, since linguistic ability is encouraged in the Illuminati.

Exercises for older youth will include games where groups compete against each other, and the older teen leads, with the help of an adult advisor. Groups that win are rewarded, groups that lose are punished. The youth are taught to leave behind the weak, or slow members. Unfit members are shot or killed, and the youth leader learns to do these tasks. They are taught to bring their unit through simulated battles with other units, and cool, cognitive logic under these conditions is rewarded. The goal is to creative cognitive leaders inside the military systems, who are dissociated from emotions under the stress of battle conditions.

The youth and their followers are taught and trained in all manner of crowd control. They will see special films, that address all possible responses to a military takeover, and the crowds' response. These situations are then acted out during exercises, and the older Youth leaders and their units are expected to deal with the different responses. The "crowd" is coached by their trainers to act in different ways.

The ultimate goal of all of this is to create an organized army of children, youth, and adults, who will know exactly what to do during the coming takeover of the world. The training that I described is going on not only in the U.S., but in every country in the world. Top training centers are located in Germany, Belgium, France, and Russia. Military trainers are often sent to these countries, to learn new techniques, then sent back to their home countries.

What to do:

It is important to realize that military alters inside are extremely hierarchical. They will often be ranked inside, with lower "foot soldiers" accountable to inside alters with increasing rank. Usually, the higher the military rank, the higher the alter will be inside the system. A soldier with no rank may not have much knowledge about, or pull, inside the system. Its only job is to blindly obey others, after years of conditioning to do this.

Ranking officers inside will often be modeled after outside perpetrators, officers, or trainers. An internal

General will often have much more knowledge than lower ranks, and should be befriended, as they can help with therapy.

It will take time, effort, and patience for both the survivor and the therapist to get to know these military officers. They are often abrupt, arrogant, and extremely hostile to therapy. They are often strongly loyal to the cult and proud of their badges, awards, and achievements that were earned through years of traumatization and hard work. They will often be reluctant to give this up, for the perceived "loss" engendered by leaving the cult.

They will also have strong programming surrounding them, including "honor/dishonor" suicidal programming (the brave, honorable soldier will die rather than betray his group, etc.). It is important to deal with the suicidal programming and intense limbic conditioning that many of these alters have been subjected to, while at the same time reasoning with the higher ranking members.

They will have photographic memory and recall of all aspects of military history. Giving them safe, appropriate, physical outlets in the daytime can let them vent off steam. These are very physically conditioned alters, who enjoy running, walking, target practice with guns and knives.

Letting them go hiking (with a safe support person), practice outdoor skills, can be helpful.

Acknowledging their importance to the survivor, and the trauma they underwent, respecting their loyalty, bravery, and appealing to their sense of honor to help the system stay safe (these alters often have a highly developed, although misguided, sense of honor) can help. Internal commendation for bravery, even an internal awards ceremony (they are used to this) for the parts that have decided to leave the cult, and protect the body, can be performed. They are used to praise and recognition for work well done, and need this motivation. They were used to getting this from the cult, but the survivor can turn the locus of control internally, instead of externally, to break bonds with the cult.

Military protectors can change their job to keeping the body safe, away from perpetrators. They can be a system's greatest asset, as they are great at "kicking butt", and are not easily frightened. They may be able to tell outside perpetrators to leave the survivor alone, and protect the survivor from outside accessing.

Allowing them to vent their feelings in therapy, in journaling, in pictures, and in collages can also help. Although higher ranking officers internally are often very dissociated from their feelings, they can begin to empathize with the others below them, who took their pain, and the brunt of the brutal, punitive experiences. They have to be willing to acknowledge that they were abused at some point, that they were deceived and used. Finding the youngest alters they were split from will help with this process. With time and good internal communication, as well as patience from both the therapist and survivor, military alters can become one of the strongest assets and allies in staying cult free.

CHAPTER EIGHT

CIA, GOVERNMENTAL, AND SCHOLARSHIP PROGRAMMING

Some systems will have internal CIA programming. Some of the methods mentioned in earlier chapters, such as brain wave programming and color coding were developed in part through funding by the CIA in the 1950's and 1960's. Military intelligence officers working in Langley, Virginia, used these government funds to conduct research on human subjects. They reported what they were learning to trainers throughout the U.S. and Europe.

CIA programming can include having alters in a system trained in different techniques of both finding a target, and studying the target without being detected. The end result of tagging the victim can include having a sexual assignation with the target, or may involve having people inside trained to assassinate a target.

These are complex programming sequences, and are put in over years of training, with periodic reinforcement. Alters may be trained to become hyper aware of their environment, and able to overhear conversations that are whispered. Internal recorders are taught to download these conversations, as well as other info. Photographic recall is emphasized, as the person will be hypnotized or put into a delta state for "downloading" information to the trainer or CIA operative.

The survivor with CIA programming will have been taught extensively how to "drop a tag" (detect anyone following them, and ditch them). This training will be begun in early childhood and built upon as the child grows older. They will often be taken into a neutral colored training room. They may be drugged, or hypnotized, usually a combination of both.

They will be shown training films of how a CIA operative works. They will be told that they are "special", "chosen", "one in a thousand" who is the only one who can do this special work. They are told that they get to be a secret agent for the CIA. The young child, having no idea who the CIA is, focuses on the fact that they have been chosen because they are special, needed, and will be eager to please. The child will be taken to a dinner party, or a drama set up by the trainer. There will be a group, anywhere from ten to sixteen people at the "party". Afterwards, the child will be questioned by the trainer extensively. Who was sitting where? What were they wearing? What color were their eyes? Their hair? Who gave the speech? What did they say? The child will be praised for correct answers, but punished, shocked if unable to recall details. This is to reinforce natural photographic memory, and assist the child with recording details. The next few times, the child's abilities will improve, as it wants to avoid punishment.

In the next level of training the child will be asked to observe, and figure out: who is the most important person in the room? Why? They will be taught body movements, and mannerisms, that give nonverbal clues away. The child may be taught to approach important adults, or an assigned target, first in role play, later in real life, and engage them in innocuous conversation while looking for information they have been clued to get. They may be taught to be innocently seductive, and will be dressed for the part. They will frequently be taught to lure the target into having intercourse with them.

An older youth, or adult, will also be taught not only how to lure a target into bed, but later how to kill them, if they are an assassination target, while they are asleep or relaxing after sexual relations. They will be taught to go through the target's belongings for any information needed by the trainer or cult leader. Often, before an assignment for an assassination, the cult member will be indoctrinated with reasons why killing the victim is a service to humanity. They will be lied to and told that they are the head of a porno ring, a pedophile, or a brutal villain. This will engage the assassin's natural anger towards the person, and will motivate them, while helping to overcome their natural moral reluctance and guilt at killing a human being.

They will be taught how to disguise themselves, with change of clothing, sex (masquerading as the opposite sex), makeup, contact lenses, and get out of the situation safely. They will be taught how to overcome interrogation techniques with extensive training and hypnosis, in case they are ever caught. They will be taught to self suicide with a pill or dagger, if they are ever apprehended, in most cases.

SUGGESTIONS

CIA programming will involve the use of sophisticated technology to reinforce its effectiveness, and can be difficult to break. It may involve the person being traumatized in isolation tanks (this will also be done with brain wave programming). It may involve sensory deprivation, sensory overload, isolation, sleep deprivation. It may involve hours of listening to repetitive tapes on headphones. The subject is shocked, or severely punished, if they try to remove the headphones. They will be hypnotized, tortured; subjected to different drug combinations; they will be exposed to harmonic tones, often in one ear or the other. They will be exposed to flashing strobe lights, which may induce a seizure, and alters will be programmed to cause seizures if the subject tries to break programming. They will be shown high speed films with different tracks, one for the left eye and one for the right eye, to increase brain splitting or dichotomous thinking.

The survivor and therapist need to work slowly to undo the effects of this trauma. The person will need to come to terms, slowly, and carefully, with how the programming was done. They may need to learn their own access codes (this will also be true of brain wave, and other sophisticated programming techniques). They will need to communicate with the traumatized alters and fragments inside, let them know they were used. They will need to help the young alters, who were split to create the system, and often underwent the worst traumas. Grieving for the abuse, the trauma, the methodical calculation used and scientific methods used to put in this programming, will take time. Venting feelings, including rage, safely will be important. The survivor may be afraid of strong feelings and will fear especially anger and rage, since they will associate those feelings with having to kill, hurt, or assassinate others. Allowing the feelings to be expressed slowly and carefully, being aware that homicidal and suicidal feelings will probably come up, is important.

If there is a concern about the ability to control acting out, the client may need to go inpatient in a safe facility that understands mind control and cult programming. They will fear being labeled "psychotic" since the programmers told them that they would be called this, and locked up forever. The WORST thing a therapist or hospital can do in a situation like this, is play into those fears, or label the person psychotic. Constant grounding in reality, using grounding exercises; slow, careful venting of rage and betrayal feelings; reinforcing over and over that the survivor can remember, and NOT go psychotic, or die, BELIEVING and VALIDATING the survivor, are all important. The survivor may have unstable behavior at points, but this is not psychosis, but rather, the natural reaction to extreme trauma. The survivor needs to realize this, and that they can overcome its effects, with time and good therapy. They will need hope, and a good support system.

GOVERNMENTAL PROGRAMMING

Governmental programming will involve the person being trained to take leadership positions or administrative positions in the government. They may be trained to network with others in governments, both local , national, and international. The Illuminati's stated goal is to infiltrate, and eventually cause the downfall of, all major governments in the world. Government operatives are taught to do this by: infiltrating local political parties running for leadership both locally and nationally working for top leaders, as administrators, financial advisors funding governmental races and backing the person sympathetic to the Illuminati, or putting their person in to win, creating political chaos and unrest with operatives trained in dissension. The people selected for governmental programming are usually highly intelligent with native charm, or charisma. They are also skilled people manipulators. These abilities may be enhanced through programming, encouraging the person to project a "persona" that will draw people to them.

They are also taught finances extensively. This programming is done by: hypnotizing the person, whether child, youth, or adult (it is usually initiated in late childhood in suitable candidates), and inducing deep trance with drugs. The person is shocked, then told the trainer's and cult agenda for the person. They are told that they are very special to the Illuminati, and will be one of the people who helps change world history. They are told they will be rewarded with wealth, popularity and power for achieving the cult's agenda. They are told, and shown, what the punishment for disobedience is. They are shown training films about government, how it works, national and international affairs. They will meet with special teachers, who coach them on the inner political workings of the group they want to infiltrate, including the power structure and strengths and weaknesses of key players.

They will learn any languages necessary for the position. They will go to University, or get any training and education needed for credibility. They will receive special scholarships to finance this, if needed.

They are given opportunities to practice their skills at infiltration, information gathering, people manipulation, and politics in set ups, and later in real situations. If they need to learn to control the media, they will learn methods to do this. They will have extensive back up and coaching during their entire career.

SUGGESTIONS

Governmental programming is quite complex, since it ties in with the person's natural abilities. They may not be able to separate themselves easily from the role that they perform and often will only feel that they are acceptable when they do their job. They may find it difficult to believe that their career, friendships, marriage and contacts have been secretly guided by the cult for most of their life. These parts may feel offended, betrayed, or furious when this realization hits. They will also find it difficult not to use the manipulation skills that come so naturally, both on their therapist, and themselves, to dull the pain that the truth may bring. The person and the alters that have undergone this type of programming have a lot to lose if they give up their roles and persona, and need to count the cost of getting out and acknowledge the difficulty of doing so. They will need to grieve over being used, and for the false interpretation of reality they have believed all their lives. Listening to other parts inside and acknowledging the reality of the cult abuse will be important steps in breaking free. Success in a new career in the person's daily life will also help restore a broken self image.

SCHOLARSHIP TRAINING

The Illuminati revere scholarship, especially oral tradition. Children with good memories and native intelligence may undergo specific training in the area of scholarship. This will include learning under trauma, with praise for accomplishment. It will also mean punishment or being shocked for poor performance. Some of the major areas of scholarship include, but are not limited to:

Oral tradition: history of the Illuminati, especially the child's particular branch, memorizing genealogies. Learning and becoming fluent in multiple languages, both modern and ancient, including but not limited to: English, French, German, Russian, Spanish, Arabic, Latin, Greek, Hebrew, Egyptian hieroglyphics; ancient Babylonian, ancient Chaldean and cuneiform writings. Some revered ancient texts are written in very ancient languages, and certain ceremonies may include rituals which utilize them. Learning ancient and modern history and becoming adept at planning role plays and dramatizations. Learning to teach others the above skills. The child who becomes adept at scholarship will also be expected to become a skilled teacher, and in turn, pass their knowledge down to others. They will practice teaching in both classroom and individual sessions.

SUGGESTIONS

Scholarship programming will involve alters who are intensely loyal to the cult, since they believe they are related to a long, unbroken line of people since earliest history. They will often be immersed in cult philosophy, having read and memorized numerous esoteric volumes related to it. Appealing to logic, intellect, having an open mind and discussing the pros and cons of leaving the cult with them will often be received the best. They despise open conflict, and prefer addressing issues intellectually. They will be skilled debaters, and quite verbal. Asking them to read books that address becoming free from the cult, and asking them to sit in and listen to accounts from traumatized alters both in their system and others inside, will often help them make the decision to switch loyalties. Although they will have been immersed in false ideologies and doctrines, they are frequently willing to attempt to be intellectually honest. They will read and debate both sides of an issue, and may become some of the first to make the decision to leave the cult once convinced that it is abusive.

CHAPTER NINE

PROGRAMMING LINKED TO STORIES, MOVIES, CARTOONS, OR ROLE PLAY DRAMATIZATION

In this chapter, I want to address a special type of programming that is universal with the Illuminati. It is programming that is linked to a story, movie, cartoon, or role play dramatization.

For countless centuries, Illuminati trainers and leaders have used role playing to reinforce as well as program children, and it is a favorite mode of teaching up to this day. A typical drama set up, or role play, will involve a "visit through time." The child is told, while drugged or hypnotized, that it and the other children with it (usually, a small group will go through this programming together) are going to " time travel". The trainer or teacher is seen as immensely powerful by the children, as he or she magically transports them through time. They enter another room, where people are dressed up in period costumes from whichever time period in history the teacher wants the children to see. Everything is historically accurate and well researched. An example: if the children are to visit ancient Rome, they will be taken to a room in the Senate, where the characters are dressed in togas. They will be speaking to each other in ancient Latin and debating issues. Caesar, or another king will enter the senate. Roman customs for a scenario such as this one will be adhered to throughout the role play.

One purpose of this role playing, is that the children are told they are getting a "behind the scenes " peek at history. Illuminati agenda will be put forward, and the children will "see" that famous figures in history were actually Illuminists. This will reinforce their "special ness" and the historicity of the group. It will also reinforce language training, since the scenes may occur in medieval England, or the French court of Louis XIV, etc. The scenes will also contain a moral that builds on programming the children have been undergoing. Maybe they will watch a "traitor" being "guillotined" in the French court. Or an unworthy senator, who tries to betray his king, will be stabbed. The child may be given a role in the play, such as taking a secret message to the king or queen, to reinforce courier programming. The child really believes that they have stepped back into history, and are part of the process of helping create history.

With modern times, programming has become more sophisticated with the advent of technology. Before television or movies, programming was often "scripted" around famous fairy tales, or stories, read aloud by one trainer while the second trainer worked with the child. A good see-song voice is necessary in a "reader". The child would be read the story, and under hypnosis and trauma, told that they are one of the characters in the story. They are told the "real" meaning of the story, its "hidden meaning" and told that whenever they hear the story, to remember what it really means.

Now days, movies and videos are frequently used in programming. Favorite scripts include: Walt Disney movies (Disney was an Illuminist), especially Fantasia, Sleeping Beauty, The Little Mermaid, Cinderella, Beauty and the Beast. The Wizard of Oz, both books and movie, has been used. Any movie that incorporates Illuministic themes can be used. E.T. and Star Wars have been used in more recent years.

HOW SCRIPT PROGRAMMING IS DONE

The trainer will play the movie for the child. The child is told that they will be "asked about " the movie, this cues the child to use photographic recall about what they are viewing. The trainer may show the child an edited shorter version of the movie, with only parts of the whole, or may show the child a short scene from the movie.

After watching the movie, or scene, the child is drugged to relax it, then asked what it remembers. The child will be shocked if it cannot recall items the trainer deems important, and will be forced to watch the scenes repetitively.

When the child has total recall of the segments, the trainer will tell the child that it is one of the characters. The child may be heavily traumatized first, and a blank slate personality created inside to be the desired character. The first thing the blank slate sees is a recording of the movie, or scene. This is its "first memory". The trainer will then link the scene with Illuminati ideology. They will teach the child the "hidden meaning" in the movie, and praise the child for being one of the few "enlightened ones" who can understand what it truly means. The script programming will often be linked to other programming the child is undergoing. Military programming may be linked to Star Wars. Total recall programming may be linked to Data in Star Trek. Computer programming may be linked to Hal in 2001 A Space Odyssey; internal labyrinth programming may be linked to the movie "Labyrinth". The possibilities are quite varied and will depend on both the child and the trainer as to which direction script programming will go. Music from the show, or scene, will be used as a trigger to access the programming inside or bring forward these personalities.

SUGGESTIONS

Scripted programming will often involve a great deal of traumatization, to create the "blank slate" alters desired. The programming will be ground in with repetition, electroshock, torture, drugging and hypnosis. The alters inside who have gone through this programming will often be highly disconnected from external reality and may believe that they are part of a "script". They may be Dorothy seeking the Emerald City (or the achievement of Illuminati rule on earth). They may be a computer or the character Data. Reality orientation will be very important. Allow these parts to experience safe outside reality, and test for themselves if they are really part of a man or woman. Looking in a mirror may help, when they express readiness. Having cognitive helpers who can share daily life memories with them, may help to ground them. At first they will be very surprised, even indignant or hostile, at suggestions that they are not the character. They will think the therapist is a trainer, or part of the script, since this is the only reality that they have known. Re-grounding, patiently, over and over to present reality, increased communication with others inside, and eventually grieving over the intense amount of trickery and deception that they experienced, will be necessary. With time and patience these parts will be willing to give up their old "scripted" roles and become part of the person's present reality.

SVALI

CHAPTER TEN

THE SIXTH STEP OF DISCIPLINE: BETRAYAL; TWINNING, INTERNAL WALLS, STRUCTURES, GEOMETRY

This chapter will address the sixth step of discipline in the Illuminati:

BETRAYAL PROGRAMMING

Betrayal programming will begin in infancy, but will be formalized at around ages six to seven, and continue on into adulthood. The sixth step can be summarized as : "betrayal is the greatest good." The Illuminists teach this to their children as a very important spiritual principle. They idealize betrayal as being the true state of man. The quick witted, the adept, learns this quickly and learns to manipulate it.

The child will learn this principle through set up after set up. The child will be placed in situations where an adult who is kindly, and in set up after set up "rescues" the child, gains its trust. The child looks up to the adult as a "savior" after the adult intervenes and protects the child several times. After months or even a year of bonding, one day in a set up the child will turn to the adult for help. The adult will back away, mocking the child, and begin abusing it. This sets in place the programming: adults will always betray a child and other adults.

Another set up will involve twinning, which deserves special mention here. The Illuminati will often create twin bonds in their children. The ideal is to have a set of real twins, but of course this is not always possible. So, the child is allowed to play with, and become close to, another child in the cult from earliest childhood. At some point early on, the child will be told that the other child is actually their "twin", and that they were separated at birth. They are told that this is a great secret and not to tell anyone, on pain of punishment. The child, who is often lonely and isolated, is overjoyed. It has a twin, someone who has a special bond to them by birth.

The children do everything together. They are taught together, do military training together. They tell each other secrets. They are also frequently friends in the daytime as well. They are taught to cross access each other just as real siblings would be.

But at some point, they will be forced to hurt each other. If one "twin" is considered expendable, the ultimate set up will be one in which one twin is forced to die while the other watches. One twin may gather secrets from the other twin, be forced to disclose them to a trainer or cult leader, then may be forced to kill the other. One twin may be forced to hit, or hurt the other. If they refuse, the other twin will be brutalized by the trainer, and the refusing twin told that the child was hurt because of their refusal to comply. Many setups will involve one twin being forced to betray the other, turning on the other child after intense programming. This betrayal set up will devastate both children, and they will learn the true lesson: trust no one. Betray, or be betrayed.

The children will also have adult role models on every hand, since the cult is a very political, hierarchical, back stabbing society. Adults are constantly betraying each other, stepping over each other to move up. The children will watch one adult being praised, advanced, because they betrayed others below them, or set them up to fail. The children will learn quickly to mimic the adults around them, and both adults and children can become quite cynical as to human nature. They will have seen it at its worst, whether in training sessions, the brutality of a C.O. in military, or the gossip and back stabbing that occurs before and after rituals. They also incorporate the message internally: play the game, or be run over. Even the youngest children learn to manipulate others adeptly, at a very young age, while the adults laugh at how quickly they are learning adult ways. People manipulation is considered a fine art in the cult, and those who do it best, as in any group, often win out.

SUGGESTIONS

Betrayal programming may have totally shattered the survivor's trust in outside people. It will take a therapist a long, long time to gain the survivor's trust. These are people who were taught over and over again that talking, sharing one's secrets, would be punished harshly. Inside littles will be very cautious at first, not trusting that the therapist is not just another trainer who will one day shout "aha!" and betray them if they begin to trust. This trust building takes time and patience, and must be earned through session after session where the therapist shows trustworthiness and non abusiveness. Survivors will test therapists over and over again, to see if they really are what they say they are. This is a normal part of the therapy process. Survivors may even try to back away from therapy, or outside support, as true caring support will "wig them out", i.e. conflict incredibly with their world view and experiences prior to leaving the cult.

Both survivor and therapist need to realize that some amount of distrust is healthy, based on what the survivor has experienced, and may be life saving, helping to protect them from outside accessing. Honor this need and be patient while the survivor tests over and over. The survivor can try to reason with inside alters who may have been betrayed to the point of legitimate paranoia. They may ask them to watch, and see what the therapist, and/or support person is like. To take their time, check them out. To be aware that what they went through may magnify normal feelings of caution. Helping orient these parts to outside reality, and especially positive experiences of trusting a little, and not being harmed, will help make great strides in undoing this. The survivor may feel confusion and internal conflict, as they experience a world where trust is possible. They may pull away, or the reverse, become highly dependent on the therapist and share too quickly due to a longing for safe intimacy that has never been met. Setting healthy boundaries while acknowledging needs will help the survivor through this stage.

Another type of programming involves the deliberate creation of internal structures within the cult member.

INTERNAL STRUCTURES: TEMPLES, EYES, MIRRORS, CAROUSELS ETC.

The Illuminati trainers will try to create internal structures within the person's personality systems. Why? They believe this creates better stability. It also gives the alters and fragments a place to "hang on to" inside, and creates a convenient way to call them up. If a fragment is indexed inside to an internal helix, for example, the trainer knows how to locate them more easily.

Internal structures will vary greatly depending on the trainer, the group, the region of the U.S. or Europe and the goals for the individual. Common internal structures will include, but are not limited to:

- **Temples:** these are often consecrated to principle Illuminati deities, and spiritual alters will congregate here. This may represent actual temples, Masonic or private, that the subject may have visited.

- **Temple of Moloch** will be created out of black stone with a fire burning internally.

- **All-seeing eye of Horus:** one of the most common structures in an Illuminati system; universal. Horus is a deity revered by the Illuminati, and the all-seeing eye internally represents the fact that the cult can always see what the individual is doing. It will also represent being given to Horus in a high ceremony. The eye may be closed, or open, depending on the system's status at the time. This eye will also be linked to demonic watching of the person's activities at all time.

- **Pyramids:** the Illuminati revere ancient Egyptian symbology, especially "mystery religion" and Temple of Set teachings. Pyramids will be placed internally both for stability (a triangle, and/or pyramid represents strength and stability), and as a calling place for the demonic. Pyramids and triangles, and the number three, represent calling up the demonic in Illuminist philosophy.

- **Sun:** represents Ra, the sun god

- **Geometric figures:** configurations of circles, triangles, pentagons, etc. Geometric patterns are considered sacred, and are based in ancient philosophy. There may be hundreds overlapping in a training grid for complex systems, which will house fragments in each one.

- **Training grids:** these may be simplistic, such as cubes with patterns on them, rows of boxes, or more complex such as helixes, double helixes, infinity loops. Each trainer will have favorites classified as simple, medium and complex, depending on the child and its ability to recall and memorize.

- **Columns:** Greek Doric, ionic columns. Often hold "time travel" programming, with a portal between two columns.

- **Computers:** complex, highly dissociated systems with alters and fragments held within a computer system.

- **Robots:** may be seen in older systems

- **Crystals:** gems, balls, multifaceted. Used in spiritual systems to enhance occult powers. Alters and fragments may congregate on facets of a large ball.

- **Mirrors:** used internally to reinforce other programming sequences, internal twinning, and distortion of reality programming. May create shadow systems of functional systems. May also lock in demonic programming.

- **Carousels:** used in some programming sequences to confuse alters inside. Often linked to spin, confusion programming internally. May be used to punish internal alters; they will be spun on the carousel if they tell.

- **Deck of cards:** this can include cards from a deck, or complex configurations made of hundreds of card inside. Dominoes programming is similar. All touch each other and if person tries to dismantle programming, the deck will "fall".

- **Black boxes:** represent self destruct and shatter programming sealed off into a black box to protect system. Should not be opened without careful preparation and good therapy.

- **Mines, booby traps:** see above

- **Spider webs:** represent linked programming, with a spider (internal programmer) who continuously reweaves the web and reinforces internal programming and punishments. The web also communicates with other systems. Can also represent demonic linkages internally, woven in.

- **Internal training rooms:** used as punishments for internal alters. Will represent external training rooms person has been in.

- **Internal walls:** these will often represent very large internal amnesia barriers. The walls may be very thick, impermeable or semi permeable. A typical use for a wall will be to maintain high levels of amnesia between "front" or daily living, amnesic alters, and "back" or cult active alters that contain more of the person's life history. The back may be able to selectively see over and cross past the wall, but the front will be completely unaware that there is a wall, or what lays behind it.

- **Seals:** usually in a group of six or seven, represent demonic sealing, and may cover end times, shatter programming, as well as role within cult in new hierarchy.

These are some common programming structures. Again, there are many, many other types of internal structures used and the number and type are only limited by the trainer's and survivor's creative abilities.

The way that these structures are placed within the person are fairly similar. Under drugs, hypnosis and electroshock, the person is traumatized into a deep trance state. In the deep trance they will be told to open their eyes and look at: either a projected image of the structure, a 3D model of it, or a holographic image using a virtual reality headset. The image will be ground in, using shock and bringing the image closer and closer to the person's visual field. It may be rotated, if graphics are available, or a 3D is used. They may be told that they are entering inside it, if it is a temple or pyramid, under deep hypnosis, that they (the alter being programmed) will now "live inside" the structure/box/card, etc. This will also be used to reinforce amnesia and isolation programming internally, since the structure will be used to reinforce walls between the alter/ fragment and other alters and fragments internally.

SUGGESTIONS

If the survivor finds structures inside, it will help for them first of all to try and realize WHY they are there. What purpose do they serve? To reinforce amnesia? Isolation? spiritual programming? punishment? To hold dangerous programming sequences? This is important, since some structures such as internal walls or barriers may have been created not only by the cult, but reinforced by the survivor as well, as a means of internal protection. The survivor may not want to dismantle internal structures too quickly without knowing their purpose and what they contain. Both the survivor and the therapist will need to go slowly. Learning how the structures were put in and which alters are linked to the structure, will be a first step. Long, slow and careful preparation, with lots of system cooperation, will be needed to look at some structures. This may only come after years of extensive therapy. Each survivor will progress at their own pace. If a wall is present, taking it down slowly, one brick at a time, or allowing part of it to become semi permeable, may be first steps in healing. Training rooms can have the equipment turned off and dismantled; it can be turned into a safe room, redecorated and refitted with toys and safe objects. Computers can slowly begin to realize that they are human, and gradually allowed to take on human characteristics.

Survivors can use their creativity to reclaim themselves, with the support of their therapists, and undo what was done.

CHAPTER ELEVEN

SUICIDAL PROGRAMMING

I have decided to write an entire chapter about suicidal programming, since it is often the most dangerous programming that the survivor will face during their healing process. ALL ILLUMINATI SURVIVORS WILL HAVE SUICIDAL PROGRAMMING PROTECTING THEIR SYSTEMS. I emphasized this to also reiterate the need for good therapy and a strong support system for the survivor.

The Illuminati know and realize that with time, individuals in their group may start to question what they are doing. Or they may become disenchanted with their role. They may even desire to leave the group or try to dismantle their own programming.

The trainers are well aware of this possibility and to prevent this, will always program in suicidality. The suicidality, or suicidal programming, may surround one or more systems internally. It may be layered into more than one system.

From earliest childhood, survivors have been conditioned to believe that they would rather die than leave their "family" (the Illuminati group). This is the core, or basis of suicidal programming. It will be closely linked to loyalty to one's family as well as the group (remember, this is a generational group and leaving it may mean giving up contact with one's parents, spouse, siblings, aunts, uncles, cousins and children, as well as close friends). These people will all try to contact the survivor, and try to draw them back into the cult, asking "don't you love us anymore?", or even becoming accusatory and hostile if the survivor does not respond the way they wish. The survivor will be told that they are "crazy". Or delusional. That their family loves them and would never be part of a cult. The family members will all still be amnesic, unless something happens to trigger their own memories.

One of the most frequent suicidal programming sequences placed internally will be "come back or die " programming. A family member may activate it by telling the survivor that they are missed and their family wants to see them. If the survivor fails to return, the programming will start running. It can only be deactivated by a code word from the person's trainer or cult contact person. This ensures that they will recontact. If the survivor tries to break this programming, they will need assistance, both internal and external, for safety.

Hospitalization may be needed in a safe facility that understands DID and programming, as well as suicidality, as the alters inside will begin fighting if the person tries to break the programming. They have been programmed to commit suicide, or be shattered internally, or at the very least, severely punished, and are afraid of the repercussions of not obeying. The survivor will need to get to know these internal alters, and reassure them that they no longer need to do their jobs.

Chronometric suicidal programming is another type placed within. This does not need contact with family members to activate. In fact, it is activated automatically after a certain amount of time WITHOUT cult contact. Controller alters and/or punishing alters will have been programmed that if a certain period of time goes without contact with the trainer, they are to commit suicide. They will be told that the only way to prevent this is recontact with the trainer, who knows a command code to halt the program. The time interval may be anywhere from three months to nine months, each system is different. Call back programming may have this type of programming as a back up, to ensure that it is followed through on.

Systems layered programming is a particularly complex form of suicide programming where several systems (up to six at a time), are programmed to fire off suicide programming simultaneously. This always needs hospitalization for the survivor's safety.

Honor/dishonor programming is common in military systems. In this, the military parts are told that an "honorable and courageous" soldier will take his life, rather than reveal secrets or leave his unit.

"No tell" programming will often be reinforced by suicidal programming.

Access denied programming, which prevents unauthorized access both externally and internally, will often be reinforced by either or both suicidal/homicidal programming.

Almost all suicidal programming is put in place to either ensure continued obedience to the cult's agenda; to ensure regular recontact; or prevent the individual or an outside person from accessing the person's system without authorization (i.e. the correct access codes, which the trainers are careful to use at the beginning of each session). It will frequently block therapy, as the survivor will be terrified, and rightly so, of dying if they reveal their internal world, or disclose their history.

SUGGESTIONS

First, both the survivor and the therapist need to find out what suicide programming is present (it's a safe bet it's there, no need to ask IF it is present). Internal communication, and finding out which alters or fragments hold suicide programming will be important. Physical safety, whether with a safe outside person, or inpatient hospitalization, while working on suicide programming is extremely important, as this programming may either drive the survivor to self destructive behavior, or back to the cult. Dealing with suicide programming assumes that the survivor and therapist have initiated good system communication internally. This is extremely important, since the survivor will need cooperation inside with dismantling suicidality.

Letting alters inside know that they no longer have to do their job, that they can change, may help. Reality orientation, letting them know that if they kill the body, that they will die, may also help (many times, these parts have been deceived into believing that they themselves will not die, if they do their jobs. This means they need to hear the truth). Having controller alters, high alters with pull inside the system, agree to help the therapist dismantle the programming will help. But be aware that SOME INTERNAL SUICIDE SEQUENCES WILL BE PUT IN THAT EVEN CONTROLLERS CANNOT DISMANTLE. Creating a safety committee inside whose main job is to keep the body safe and ask for help if suicidal programming begins to kick in, BEFORE ACTING OUT OCCURS, will also help tremendously.

As the survivor develops trust with their therapist and realizes the value of life, and that life can be much better than it has ever been before, they will become more willing to reach out and ask for help if they become suicidal. The survivor may also find that they encounter core despair. This despair may have been used by the cult to run suicidal programming, but it is not programming itself. A very young core split may have taken many of the feelings of despair, hopelessness, failure to thrive and desire to die, that the child felt growing up in a horribly abusive atmosphere. This is not programming but true feelings, and it will be important to differentiate this from programming. If core despair comes up, the alter containing this may also report having been trained to NOT SUICIDE, or give up. The trainers will do this, if despair begins overwhelming the subject at an early age, to prevent the child's suicide.

The survivor's cognitives, helpers, nurturers, will all need to be gathered together to help this part of the core heal. There will be intense, and rightful, grieving and anguish for the immense pain that the young child suffered. Hopelessness will come out. It can help if alters with happier memories can try and share their memories with this very young part. External support and caring can also make a big difference. Healing the immense pain held by this core split will take a long period of time and should not be hurried. Antidepressants can help, as the depression may be shared through all systems. Messages of hope, new and positive experiences can all help the survivor work through this type of programming, as well as journaling, poetry, artwork and collaging the feelings. Time, patience, support, the ability to vent feelings in a safe manner and physical safety when needed, will all help immensely as the survivor works through these issues.

CHAPTER TWELVE

PREVENTING REACCESSING OF THE SURVIVOR

This is by far one of the most important chapters I have written in this book. Why? Deprogramming cannot be consistently successful if the person is still in contact with the abusers.

Survivors will take one step forward, then will find themselves knocked down internally. All the hard work in therapy will be undone or set back. They and their therapist will find that they have trouble finding internal alters. Whole systems may shut down. A child presenting system may come out.

Confusers and scramblers will take over therapy sessions and blockers will block therapy.

No one chapter can ever be totally comprehensive in how to prevent reaccessing. What I will share are some of the more common ways that the cult and trainers will try to reaccess individuals, and give some techniques on avoiding this.

The cult has a vested interest in keeping its members. After all, it has spent generations telling its members that if they leave they will die, be killed, or go psychotic. It makes them quite unhappy to see someone who is quite alive and very clearly not psychotic leave. It also makes their more restive members question the truth of what they have been told if they see someone get out. Having a member leave may break the hold of some programming in other members. Trainers especially hate to see anyone leave, and grind their teeth over this problem at night. People leaving the cult is considered a training failure and the trainers may be punished severely.

So, the cult has come up with certain ways to keep their members with them, willingly or unwillingly. These include, but are not limited to:

E.T. phone home (phone programming) : the individual will have personalities whose sole job is to call and report to the trainer or cult leader. These are often young child alters who are eager to please, starved for attention and nurture, and who are heavily rewarded for calling back in. Any survivor who attempts to leave the cult must deal with the urge to phone home. To phone their abusers. To phone their friends who are in the group. To phone their parents, siblings, cousins, or aunts. This urge may become overwhelming at times and worst of all, the survivor may be totally amnesic to the fact that the people they are calling are cult members who are urging them, in code, to come back. Common phrases used include: your 'family' loves you, misses you, needs you. So and so is ill and needs to see you. You are so special to us. You are so valuable. You need to come see us. Why are you so distant? Why haven't we heard from you lately?

The list goes on and on. Sweet, kind phrases with double meanings, placed in the person during training sessions. Trainers are not stupid and know that if cult members said "come to the ritual meeting at midnight next week", the survivor would run the other way, and be validated as well that they are not making things up. So, they ingrain code messages behind innocuous phrases such as described above.

These, and other messages, are meant to trigger recontact programming.

In recontact programming, (ALL ILLUMINATI MEMBERS HAVE RECONTACT PROGRAMMING, IT IS NEVER LEFT TO CHANCE) the person has parts whose only job is to have contact with their trainer or cult leader, or accountability person (person one step above them in the cult). These parts are heavily programmed under drugs, hypnosis, shock, torture, to have recontact. The individual will feel restless, shaky, weepy, afraid if they try to break this programming. It will often be linked or joined in to suicidal programming (see previous chapter for more on suicidal programming). They may experience PTSD symptomology, or even flood programming, and internal self punishment sequences, as they fight this programming internally.

Siblings are often cross trained to access each other with special codes. Remember when.... may initiate this. I love you, or, your family loves you, can also be used. Phrases will be individual, depending on the person's family members and background.

Certain clothing or jewelry worn can be used to draw a cult loyal system, such as a color coded system, or jewel system , to the front. The person must physically resemble the person the individual was "keyed into" during the programming sequence, to prevent inadvertent popping out of alters by anyone wearing a ruby pin, for example. This kind of cueing will be based on sight recognition of a person, plus the clothing color or jewelry being worn a certain way.

Phone calls from concerned family members, friends, and cult members will flood the survivor's phone lines and answering machine, especially during the initial getting out phase.

Hang up calls, three or six in a row, or calls where a series of tones are heard, may be used as cues to recall the individual and fire off internal programming.

Birthday, holiday or we miss you cards, or letters, may be sent with trigger codes imbedded in them.

Flowers with a certain number of flowers, or color may be sent. Daisies may fire off daisy programming internally.

The possibilities are almost endless, depending on the trainers, the group the person was with, and the people they are most bonded to in the cult. Special training sessions will be given, with code words and cues built into the system's programming.

If all else fails, hostility will start. "You don't love us" will be heard, even when the survivor has stated repeatedly that they care. Boundaries drawn with cult members will be misinterpreted as lack of concern, or withdrawal. Accusations, guilt, and anger as well as manipulation will be used as hooks to make the survivor feel guilty for withdrawing from the cult.

Isolation programming may activate, as the cult support system is withdrawn in the survivor's life, and they try the difficult task of developing healthy, appropriate relationships outside of the cult. Often, the therapist will be the survivor's lifeline and sole support at first. The individual may fall into codependent relationships quickly, or relationships with other survivors to fill the void in their life. At worst, desperate for caring and feeling isolated, they will make friends with the first kind person they meet. This person could be a cult set up, sent to initiate a friendship quickly. Survivors should be wary of "instant friendships" or instant bonding with others. Most good relationships take time and effort.

SUGGESTIONS

One of the most difficult tasks, but most important safety wise, will be for a totally amnesic presenting system to realize who their abusers really are. It will seem unbelievable, when back parts come up in therapy, and disclose that beloved, or even barely tolerated family members are in the cult. Believing these parts and listening to them will be crucial to safety. Protectors will be important to the survivor's safety, especially if they are willing to give up cult allegiance and help keep the person safe. Outside accountability with safe persons is extremely important. The problem is that generational Illuminati survivors have often been surrounded all their lives by a network of other cult members. Unknown to them, their closest friends and family members are part of the group. Amnesia poses the greatest danger to the survivor in the beginning stages, as they will trust people before they remember that they are unsafe.

A survivor may remember the father taking them to rituals, and believe that their mother or grandparent is safe. Only later in therapy will they remember that mother or granny was actually their trainer, since the most painful memories tend to come later. The survivor may only remember ritual abuse in early childhood, and think they were let go at a certain age. This is extremely rare, since the group has put in years of effort into training them. Almost never will they just "let someone go" in generational families. But they may be given false or screen memories, especially if they are in therapy, to confuse the survivor and the therapist.

The client will need to listen to and believe internal parts who have more information than they do, and take appropriate steps to be safe. This will probably mean cutting off contact with perpetrators at this point. Again, outside accountability is paramount. Safe houses, a women's shelter or a safe church family may be alternatives. One of the worst things the survivor can do is isolate, or go out walking late at night alone, or go camping in the woods by themselves. Abduction will often occur in these scenarios, when the survivor is alone and vulnerable. Safe roommates can help keep the survivor safe.

Locking up the phone in the trunk of the car may help if phone programming is intense. This gives the survivor the chance to wake up or stop phone calls, if an alter has to get up, find the car keys, turn on the light, go outside, and open a car trunk, bring the phone inside and hook it up again before making a phone call.

Building a support system through safe support groups, a good therapist, church, or work can also help. Whenever possible and practical, moving away from the town or state where the survivor was active in the cult can help. Why? Remember the survivor's whole support network was the cult in their old town. The trainers and/or family members have invested time and effort into the survivor and have a big stake in their coming back. If the survivor moves far enough away, a cult group in the new city or state will not know them as well, and will not have a lengthy history with them. This can help decrease the chance of reaccessing by the cult, in conjunction with good therapy and a safe support network.

The survivor will have to rebuild their support system anyway, so why not do it as far as possible away from people they have known who might hurt them? It can be intensely triggering to the survivor to see their old trainer walking down the street towards them, and inside alters may destabilize or feel unsafe. This is one case where distance is good.

One caution though: even if the survivor moves, they will need to work intensely on blocking internal recontact programming at the same time, or they may be quickly reaccessed. Trainers will often send the person's system codes and grids over the internet to cult groups in the new city, and will try to send someone who physically resembles the trainer or a family member to initiate contact with the survivor.

Internal communication and letting inside alters know that they can change their jobs will help. Reward internal reporters for changing allegiance and committing to keep the survivor safe. The cult used to reward them for doing their job; now the survivor can reward them for changing jobs. Develop new interests, work or hobbies that can help the survivor meet new, safe people. The survivor may want to practice friendship skills in support groups, as long as they are run by reputable, safe therapists.

Be aware that holiday dates are often important dates for reaccessing. Calendars are available that show important holidays for SRA groups. Birthdays are also dates when the individual is expected to return and there may be programming surrounding this.

Callback programming (where the person is given a specific date or holiday when they are to return to the cult, or be punished) may need to be broken as well. Allowing the alters who went through the programming to share their memories, acknowledging their needs, and trying to meet those needs in healthy ways will bring healing.

The survivor will need to go through a period of grieving for loss of contact with family members and friends in the cult. No matter how abusive, how disliked, it can be very difficult to cut off with perpetrators, especially if they were the only people close to the survivor. The survivor needs to acknowledge the difficulty of creating a new, healthy, cultless support group. The survivor needs to recognize that learning new skills and developing healthy friendships will take time.

One issue often brought up by survivors is: how much do I tell others about my past? This is an individual decision that the survivor and therapist need to look at together. In general though, caution in sharing is best, since sharing too much about the survivor's past may draw the wrong people to them.

These people may be dysfunctional, or possible cult members. It is usually best to base new, non cult friendships on healthy aspects of the person at first and very gradually share small bits of information as the friendship progresses, and sharing seems appropriate. With time and opportunities, the survivor will learn the importance of appropriate boundaries and will want healthier relationships in their life.

CHAPTER THIRTEEN

SHELL PROGRAMMING, INTERNAL COUNCILS, HUMAN EXPERIMENTATION, FUNCTION CODES

Parts of this chapter could be extremely triggering, please read with caution and only with a therapist if a survivor.

Shell programming is a form of programming used to create a "shell" on the outside, that other alters inside speak through. This is a designed to hide the person's multiplicity from the outside world, and works extremely well with highly fragmented systems. It also takes a person with the ability to dissociate to a great degree.

How it is done: with shell programming, the trainer will often take a clear plastic or glass mask, and put it in front of the subject. They will be extremely traumatized, shocked, drugged, and told that they (the alter or alters in front) are the "mask" that they see. Their job will be to be a shell, or voice, to cover for the others behind. These parts will be so traumatized that they literally see themselves as only a shell, with no real substance or body.

Others inside will then be directed to come next to the "shell" alters, and use their voice to cover their own. This allows greater fragmentation of the person, while being able to hide it from outside view, since the internal alters will learn to present through the shell. Shell alters always see themselves as "clear", and will have no color if color coding is present in other systems.

SUGGESTIONS

It is important to realize that what the system is actually doing is co-presenting, although not co- consciously. For a shell program to work, the shell alters have been taught to allow co-presentation with the other alters in the systems. Other alters in the back may not always be aware that this is what is happening, and the front shell especially will not know that they are being "gone through" for co-presentation.

Recognizing the trauma that occurred, and finding out where the shell fragments came from, will help. Allowing both the shell alters and the other alters to recognize that this is how they have been presenting, and why, will be an important step. Back alters may then begin presenting without going through the shell, and the person may look "more multiple" than they ever have for a period, with accents or young voices coming through. What is actually happening is that the back is presenting without masking who they are through the shell. Meanwhile, the shell alters may decide to coalesce, for greater strength, and may decide to change jobs. Each system will decide what is best for them.

INTERNAL COUNCILS

Survivors of Illuminati programming will always have some type of hierarchy inside. This is because the cult itself is very hierarchical, and puts this hierarchy inside the person. What better way to inspire loyalty to leadership than to put the leadership inside the person's head? Trainers are also very hierarchy conscious themselves. They know that a system without hierarchy and head honchos inside to direct things will be a system in chaos. They will not leave the person's system leaderless inside.

Many trainers will put themselves in the person, over the internal programmers or trainers. This is because they are egotistical, but also because it uses a well known phenomenon of human nature: PEOPLE TEND TO INTERNALIZE THEIR ABUSERS. The survivor may be horrified to find a representative of one of their worst perpetrators inside, but this was a survival mechanism. A tenet of human behavior is that often people will punish someone less who mimics them. A brutal nazi will be less likely to punish another brutal nazi, but will look down upon and punish a weak, crying person. So, the survivor will internalize the rough nazi inside, to avoid being hurt. The survivor may mimic accents, mannerisms, even claim the perpetrator's life history as their own.

The ultimate form of internalization comes with internalizing hierarchical councils. The person, under pain, hypnosis, and drugs, will be taught to incorporate a highly dissociated group inside to lead the others. These will often be created from core splits, because the trainers want them to be extremely strong, stable alters in the system.

Triads of three elders may be seen Platinum's may have a head council of three

Jewels will have a triad, made up of ruby, emerald, diamond in many systems, to rule over the others

And, of course, an internal "leadership council", "System Above", "Ascended Masters", "supreme council", regional council, world council, etc. may be found. The councils found will vary with each survivor.

These internal groups will correlate roughly to the outside group. Often the child or youth at age twelve will be presented to these groups in a formal coming of age ceremony. This ceremony is considered quite an honor, and will involve the child being traumatized and accepting the leadership of the council for the rest of their life. Undying loyalty is promised. There may be other occasions the person will be forced to come before the councils throughout their lifespan, either for judgment, to pass tests, for punishment, or elevation. These councils will be seen as holding power of life or death, and the child or youth will do anything to gain their favor. The child will internalize them. The trainer will help with the internalization, using photographs or holographic images of the people to "burn them in". Each member of the group will be given different leadership tasks.

It is not uncommon for the survivor to incorporate a parent, both parents, or grandparents, into their internal leadership hierarchy in a generational survivor.

High priests and priestesses may sit on ruling councils inside. Suggestions:

Internal leadership councils will often be some of the most resistant to, and hostile towards therapy, especially in the early stages. They will verbally banter with, or refuse to speak to, the therapist, as being "beneath their notice." They are mimicking the haughty, hierarchical attitudes they have been exposed to all their lives.

They also have the most to lose, if the survivor leaves the cult, and may fight this decision tooth and nail. They will often be the alters with an "attitude".

Both the survivor and therapist need to recognize that these parts had powerful needs that were met in the cult setting. To ignore this and argue with them will only entrench their belief that therapists are stupid and unknowing people. Acknowledge their internal role while gently pointing out reality. Try to enlist their aid in helping the survivor strengthen. Discuss honestly the pros and cons of leaving the cult. These are highly intellectual alters, and they need to express their concerns and doubts. Setting good boundaries and not allowing verbal abuse of the therapist is important. These alters are used to "pushing people around" verbally, and have been rewarded for it prior to therapy. Now, they need to learn new coping skills and behaviors, and the process may take time. Allow them to vent their anger, displeasure, and fears about the decision to leave the cult. Offer them new jobs inside the person of leadership over safety committees, or even decision making committees.

Sometimes, a system that has broken free from the cult, and has no external hierarchy that they are accountable to will go through a short period of chaos as word gets out: we're free, and don't have to do what the cult tells us to do any more! Hundreds of internal arguments may break out as to: what do we do for a living? where do we live? what do we eat? what hobbies will we have? Everybody wants to come out, see the daytime, and live this new, free life. But the freedom may cause imbalance with all of the switching going on inside. Enlisting the aid of the internal hierarchy, and creating a limited democracy, with ground rules, may help during this time. Don't dismantle the internal hierarchy overnight, or the systems will be rudderless. Enlist their aid in helping direct which direction the survivor goes. Things will settle down after a period, as the systems learn to listen to each other, vote on ideas, and begin going together in the same direction.

HUMAN EXPERIMENTATION

This is one of the most grievous things that still occurs in the Illuminati today. The Illuminati were famed for deciding years ago to "go scientific" and incorporate scientific experimentation into their training principles. This is one area where they broke with other, more traditional groups, who still followed "spiritual principles". The Illuminati decided to use scientific data, especially in the psychiatric and behavioral sciences, to drive their training practices. This became known openly during W.W.II, when the world heard about the experimentation on Jews and other groups in the concentration camps, but human experimentation had been quietly going on for years before underground.

It also did not stop at the end of the war. German trainers and scientists were scattered around the world, and hidden, where they continued teaching others the principles they had learned, and continued with ongoing experimentation.

Some of this experimentation occurred with government funding through groups such as the CIA and NSA. The Illuminati had people infiltrated throughout these groups, who used the principles discovered and shared them with their own trainers.

Experimentation is going on, even to this day. It is done secretly. Its purpose is to help improve and create more sophisticated training techniques. To prevent "programming failures", or "pfs" as they are called in the cult.

Many, many survivors, if not all, will have been told that they are only an experiment. This may or may not be true. Trainers like to tell their subjects that they are experiments, even if they aren't, for several reasons:

1. It creates immense fear and helplessness in the subject (the thought is, if this is an experiment, I will have to work really hard to survive this)
2. It devalues the person immensely. They will feel that they have no real value as a human being, that all they are is an experiment. Someone who feels devalued doesn't care, and will be willing to do things they wouldn't if they felt some value, some humanization.
3. It gives the trainer added power, as they are the one who can begin or stop the "experiment". Almost always, when the person is TOLD they are an experiment, it isn't really true. When trainers and cult

members really do experiments, the subjects are never told, because it could bias results. The fear could interfere with drug effects, and skew the results. Most recent cult experimentation has been in the area of: drug effects: using different drugs, both alone and in new combinations and dosages, to induce trance states and open the person to training. Drugs are looked for which will shorten the time interval needed to induce trance state, which are quickly metabolized, and leave no detectable residues the next day.

Behavioral science: watching and recording data on different environmental parameters on human behavior. Modifying the environment.

PRAISE AND PUNISHMENT AS MOTIVATORS

Isolation techniques: recording data both physiological and psychological from different isolation methods. Removing, adding, combining different methods of sensory isolation, and the effect of each.

Effectiveness of virtual reality in implanting programming.

Effectiveness of new disks created to put programming in. Cult graphics and computer experts will work to create better and more effective VR disks, which are tested on cult subjects for their effectiveness. The cult wants more and more standardization, and less room for human error and weakness, in its training techniques, which is why it is going more and more to high tech equipment and videos. Attempts to break programming, cause program failure; recording what is effective, what isn't and develop new sequences to prevent pf. Subjects under hypnosis are ordered to try and break certain internal programming sequences. The ways they go about this, and what seems effective, are shared with the trainers, who then create new programs to prevent degradation of programming from occurring.

Harmonic/light, sensory deprivation and over stimulation and the effects neurologically and physically. New combinations of sensory input are always being tested to see which achieve the most lasting results, and can be done rapidly.

The cult is always trying to find new, better, faster methods to break down subjects, put programming in, and prevent the programming from failing.

This has been the emphasis in most research it has done. The results of this research is shared worldwide, both by internet, phone calls, and international trainer conferences, where trainers worldwide share the results of what they are finding. New techniques are incorporated by other groups which are eager to find out what is being discovered.

SUGGESTIONS

If you have experimental programming, realize that the alters who were used in it are heavily traumatized. They also will feel devalued, less than human, and this was reinforced heavily by the trainers who worked with them. They probably weren't used in initial experiments, as described above, but may have been used in second level experimentation.

I will explain what those terms mean.

Top trainers and leaders will initiate an experiment with a new drug. They will learn to triturate dosages, and record all observable facts on hundreds of subjects. After enough data is gotten, they will then clear it for use by trainers in local groups. It will then still be considered experimental, but will be second level, instead of first level experimentation. At this point, all trainers in local groups will be told to record and report any adverse reactions to the drug, any usual dosages needed, etc. This data is collected in databanks (yes, the cult is now in the computer age), inside of encrypted files, which will then be sent to a central base in Langley, Virginia.

Alters used in experiments, or told that they were experiments, need to realize they are valuable. They will need to realize they went through intense programming, and be allowed to vent and discuss their experiences. The fear related to believing they were an experiment needs to be vented appropriately. They will be angry at the dehumanization, intentionality, and coldness of what they went through, and quite rightly so. They may rail against the effects in their life now of the experiments and procedures they went through, and need to grieve over loss of body image; loss of trust in people; the sense of betrayal and helplessness that they felt during the procedures. They may want to journal, or draw pictures of their experiences.

A warm, empathetic therapist, who listens, and believes, and does not discount what they went through, is invaluable at this point. Allowing internal cognitives and helpers ground parts who went through bizarre sensory experiences, and creating "grounding committees" inside will also help. Extra support may be needed while dealing with experiences and feelings of this intensity.

FUNCTION CODES

Trainers will place within the subject's systems a special way to organize the fragments that are related to the job they were trained to do. These are called Function Codes, and there are three main types:

Command Codes: these are irreversible commands, put in at the limbic level of conditioning. The first code always put in is the "halt" command, which stops the person in their tracks, and is the first code any new trainer learns. This will stop the subject from assassinating their trainer, if they have MK ULTRA or other assassin training in place.

Other command codes will include: system destruct codes (suicide); shatter codes; erasure codes; and antisuicide codes.

Access Codes: these are specialized codes, often coded into short messages, or numerical codes, that allow access into the person's system. A trainer will always begin a session by repeating the person's personal complete access code, which will allow authorized entry into the system without setting off booby traps and internal protectors. These codes may also depend and be set up on sight recognition and voice recognition of the person giving the codes. In other words, the system will respond to the codes only if a person who appears to be an authorized person, such as the person's trainer, gives them. This is to prevent unauthorized access or using of the person by others outside of the person's local cult group.

Function codes: these are the "job codes" or work codes within the system.

Often, several will be coded to link together to perform a task. These are usually a letter, such as a Greek alphabet letter, combined with a numeric sequence that corresponds to their place on the internal grid or landscape.

SUGGESTIONS

If the survivor has function codes, or the other codes internally, it will help if the different system controllers can share these with the person. The person can then get to know the fragments, hear their history, and help them begin coalescing with other parts internally. It may help to find the template these codes were fragmented from, and help the template realize how they were traumatized to create these fragments.

About deprogrammers: Often people who call themselves deprogrammers will attempt to find these codes and help the person. This is an individual decision of each survivor and therapist. There may be excellent deprogrammers, but I have always felt extreme caution, and never used one myself for two reasons:

1. I would never ever give away the locus of control away to an outside person again. It would remind me to much of my own abuse, and I believe the survivor should be self empowered in therapy as much as possible.
2. There are no quick cures, or miracles, or short cuts in the process of undoing the extensive amount of abuse that has occurred with Illuminati programming. Even the best deprogrammers will admit that after they are done, the person will usually have an idea of what was put in them, but must finish with years of therapy dealing with how they FEEL about the programming that was done. Illuminati programming takes YEARS to put in, with extensive, methodical abuse, and a realistic therapist will realize that it will take years of patience, support, and hard work by both therapist and survivor to undo a lifetime of conditioning and pain. This is not to say that deprogrammers don't help people; good, reputable, safe ones have been reported to be of great help. But the person can also undertake the process themselves of undoing their own programming, and often the survivor is the best "internal deprogrammer" of all. They know their inside people and what motivates them, better than anyone else.

CHAPTER FOURTEEN

SPIRITUAL PROGRAMMING

Note: this chapter includes discussion of both cult and Christian spirituality; do not read if these themes are triggering***

Any discussion of Illuminati programming would be lacking if it did not address spiritual programming. Most of the previous chapters have dealt with scientifically based, organized, structured programming.

But the Illuminati are first and foremost not scientists, but spiritual. The very foundation of the group is based on the occult. And they go to great lengths to grind in these occult beliefs in their people's systems.

The amount of spiritual programming in the person's systems will vary from person to person, and depends on the individual group, their religious heritage, the leader's beliefs, and the trainers in the group.

All children go to rituals, where they are dedicated from before birth as well as at intervals throughout their life. In these rituals, demonic entities are invoked, to coerce the person into servant hood, loyalty, and secrecy; as well as reinforce the programming being done.

Trainers will invoke demonic layering during programming sessions. This is done after acute trauma. The person is asked if they want more pain, and they will always say “no”. The trainer then offers them a way out: if they will accept a “protector” or “protectors” they won’t be hurt any more. The trainers will want this, knowing that with these “protectors’” they can shorten the training sessions. The protectors, or guardians, will reinforce the programming internally, without outside help. This concept will seem controversial to people who do not believe in spiritual realities, but I am only describing what the Illuminists believe, and their trainers practice.

Spiritual programming will also include: being forced to memorize rituals, THE BOOK OF ILLUMINATION, and other books which contain cult beliefs. The person will be saturated from infancy on, in classes and training sessions, with cult beliefs. They will go to rituals where the adults participate in spiritual worship, wearing robes, and giving obeisance to the group’s particular guardian deity. Moloch, Ashtaroth, Baal, Enokkim are demons who are commonly worshipped. The child may see a sacrifice, either real or a set-up, to these deities; animal sacrifices are common. The child will be forced to participate in the sacrifices, and will have to go through blood baptism.

They will be forced to take the heart, or other internal organs, out of an animal that has been sacrificed, and eat them. The adults, and leaders of the group, will place their hands on the child’s head, while it is drugged, and invoke demonic entities.

One ritual which is actually programming is the "resuscitation ritual". In this ritual, the child may be heavily drugged, and shocked or tortured, to the point that his heart may stop. The head priest will then "resuscitate" the child, using drugs, CPR, and incantations. When the child comes back, and is awake, he or she will be told that they were "brought back to life" by the demonic entity that the particular group worships, and that now the child owes it their life. They are told that if they ever tell, or try to get the demon to leave, they will return to the lifeless state they were in prior to resuscitation.

Spiritual "healings" due to the demonic are also common. Injuries caused by torture, or programming sessions, or even military exercises, will be healed almost instantaneously during invocations.

Jewel programming will often have demons loyal to the generational family spirits layered in. These are called the "family jewels". The demons "guard them" and help protect the programming surrounding them.

In a sense, every ritual that a young child is part of, is an intense programming experience, as the child observes the adults around them, and imitates their behavior. The child will be severely punished if it falls asleep, and will be told that demons will kill it if it goes to sleep again during a ritual.

They are taught to be completely silent, no matter what they witness during the rituals. The child will witness things that seem utterly unbelievable, including faces appearing transformed by the demonic, channeling, other voices coming out of a leader's mouth, reading of members, telling the future. Group guidance will often be given through channeling of a strong spirit or principality; members who can channel powerful spirits and survive are respected, and their guidance will be looked for.

Some groups will use scriptures negatively or program the child to hate Christian symbols and theology. Other groups will encourage the amnesic front to embrace a Christian lifestyle, while forcing the back alters to renounce and blaspheme the choices the front has made, to separate the two alter groups even further. The cult alters will be told that since they renounced Christianity, they have committed the "unpardonable sin" and can never be forgiven. They will be shown scriptures that supposedly back this up.

In moments of despair, during intense torture or isolation, a person will often cry out to God for help. The trainers or other cult members will often mock the person, telling the person that God has forgotten them, or ask "where is God now? He must hate you....."

Any negative experience the person undergoes, will be used to reinforce the concept that they have been abandoned by God. The cult will gleefully point out the contradictions between what the person experiences, and what Christianity teaches should happen to them.

They may distort scriptures, or use false scriptures. They may distort Christian hymns, or use them in programming. A favorite hymn is "may the circle be unbroken", since it can have two meanings.

SUGGESTIONS

Spiritual programming can be some of the most damaging programming within a person's systems, since it attempts to cut them off from the source of real healing. It is an intentional distortion of truth, with events calculated to teach and reinforce wrong concepts of God. Many survivors are unable to hear Christian terms, or are intensely triggered by any religious discussion.

The survivor and therapist need to realize that these negative reactions are the result of years of false teaching, pain, punishment, distortion and set-ups. It is important not to judge the parts of the person that are negative towards spirituality, or come out, proclaiming the power and benefits of cult spirituality.

The survivor's front may be horrified to hear or learn about parts that have these feelings, especially if they are a strong Christian. These parts inside are sharing the only reality they have ever known, and need time and patience to ground, and experience reality outside of the cult setting.

Demonic oppression may need to be dealt with, and even deliverance, to bring relief to a system that is being terrorized by the demonic.

Each therapist and survivor will need to come to terms with their own spiritual beliefs. I personally believe that a therapist needs to consider the possibility of the demonic, since this is what the survivor has been exposed to all their life. The cult certainly does believe it is real, and anyone who has been involved in a cult setting will have had experiences that are in-explainable by normal rational scientific principles.

The survivor needs hope, and healing. A positive spirituality based on love, gentleness, forgiveness, that is the opposite of the coercing, punitive, negative spirituality the survivor has known, will help immensely in the healing process. A spiritual belief system that offers hope, healing, grace, mercy, and affirmation will often give the survivor the support they need to go on during the often difficult process of healing.

CHAPTER FIFTEEN

CORE SPLITS, DENIAL PROGRAMMING, THE LAST FIVE STEPS OF DISCIPLINE

VIRTUAL REALITY PROGRAMMING

Virtual reality programming (VR) is a form of programming that has become more and more widely used in the past few decades. It involves the person being placed in VR headsets and suit while a cult created VR disk is used to run the program. It can be used to create 3D and holographic images, and especially is useful in scripted programming, and target practice sequences for assassin training. Under hypnosis, the person will really believe they are in the scene.

Virtually any scenario can be recreated. Images to be "burned in" will be shown on the VR disk, and reinforced repetitively during the programming sequence. Some trainers feel it removes the element of "human error" in training, and use it quite extensively. VR programming, like any other programming, means going inside and finding out the distortions that were placed in the parts that went through the programming, allowing them to see how they were deceived, and dealing with the trauma associated with the programming.

DENIAL PROGRAMMING

Denial programming begins with the first experiences the infant goes through in life. The child has been horrendously wounded and traumatized, yet the next morning, the adults around him are acting normally, as if nothing had happened. They are modeling a lifestyle of denial for the infant and young child. This is reinforced later by the child being told:

"It was just a bad dream" (oh, how the child wants to believe this lie. It makes the pain less to think it didn't really happen)

"It's just your imagination; it isn't really happening" (which is again embraced as an escape from the horror). Denial will also be fed by the adults around the child telling them that they will never be believed if they disclose. There will be set ups to teach the child what they see and hear, and to teach the child to trust outside adults to tell them their reality.

A typical set up will go like this:

The adult will hold an object such as an orange in their hand, and ask the young child, about age two or three, "what is this?" The child will quickly respond, "oh, an orange!" The child will be shocked, and told, "no, it's an apple." The child will be confused, because what they are looking at is obviously an orange. It is the color orange, smells like an orange, looks like an orange. The question will be repeated. The child may answer again," an orange," and will be shocked again. Finally, the child, unsure and not wanting to be punished, will say, "an apple," and be praised.

The purpose of this exercise is to teach the child to not trust their own reality, and look to outside adults or leaders to tell them what reality really is.

That is the basis of denial: the person learns to not trust their own reality, because of punishment and fear when they have spoken the truth.

Alters will be created as the child grows, whose purpose is to deny the cult abuse. If any leakage or breakthrough occurs, the denial alter's job is to create a plausible explanation: it was a nightmare, a book the person read, a movie they saw, etc. These alters will read and quote literature that refutes SRA. THESE ALTERS OFTEN BELIEVE THAT THEY ARE SAVING THE LIFE OF THE SURVIVOR.

They have been told that if the survivor remembers, and believes the abuse, the survivor will be killed, or the denial alter will be severely punished or shattered for not doing their job. These parts have a vested interest in their job: they believe their very existence and they body's survival, depend upon them.

SUGGESTIONS

Arguing with a denial alter will not work, since they are not motivated by logic, but fear. A better approach is to ask them what they fear if the person remembers. This will open up the deception and lies that were ground in. They may be protecting the survivor from suicidal alters behind them, who are programmed to kick in if denial is broken through. Allowing them to vent their concerns, and enlisting the aid of helpers or cognitives who do not have suicidal or denial programming will help. Showing them reality in a gentle way, allowing them to "listen in" on others who share will go a long way.

Some denial is the natural consequence of self protection from the horrors of abuse; not all denial is programming. But if denial is constantly blocking therapy, and causing it to come to a complete standstill; if the person becomes highly suicidal every time denial is set aside briefly, then the possibility needs to be considered. Safety, inner cooperation, and patience will go a long way in decreasing denial. As denial backs down, you can expect an immense amount of grieving as the truth is realized. Denial protected the survivor from the horrendous pain of the truth, and should be let go of extremely slowly and cautiously, with plenty of support during the grieving stage.

CORE SPLITS

Core splits are intentional traumatic splits created from the core personality.

The core may be literally "splintered" by overwhelming psychological and physical/spiritual trauma. The trauma needed to create a core split must be very early and psychologically devastating. Fetal splits may occur, but they are rarely a core split; instead, the core creates an alter, but remains.

Core splits are done between the ages of 18 months and three years. Usually at least one parent or main caretaker is involved in the trauma, because this creates the psychological devastation necessary to split the core. Physical trauma alone rarely causes core splits. The torture is intense and prolonged, until the child collapses. It may be shocking, stretching, being hung in a high place, or a combination of several techniques. Being placed in "shock boxes", or near drowning are also used.

The techniques that create core splits are also dangerous, since they can also cause autism if the child cannot endure the programming. When I was in the cult, I fought to stop core splitting because occasionally children were lost or the foundational personality was too weakened.

The core may split into two, three, or up to eight splits internally. Each split will be a piece of the "core child". The original core will not resurface after splitting. These splits are used by cult trainers to be used as templates to create systems within the child. A core split, or a split from one, will be a strong alter, and can be re-split many times in the programming process, to create a multifaceted and diverse system within.

SUGGESTIONS

Core splits represent intense foundational trauma. They will be the basis for later systems, which may be completely dissociated from the split as time goes on. Work on core splits should go very slowly, and only late in the therapy process when there is immense intrasystem cooperation. The survivor will need every internal resource to deal with these traumas, and plenty of outside therapeutic support.

It may mean hospitalization unless the survivor can keep the trauma from emerging too quickly, and the therapist and survivor can go extremely slow.

Other, less dissociated systems and fragments should be integrated.

Acknowledging the abuse cognitively will be the first step in dealing with core trauma. Letting more dissociated parts grieve about "hearing about" what happened may come next. Allowing feelings near the core to come close, a little at a time, with helpers and internal nurturers offering support will help.

These feelings should be titrated, and looked at a little at a time. Splits may be different ages, and may need to express themselves in different ways.

There may be "dream programming", a "fantasy world", or other flight from reality surrounding the core splits, that protects them from contact with the outside world, which is perceived as brutal and cold.

Parts may be completely disconnected from outside reality in an effort to buffer pain.

Slow, patient nurturing and reality orientation will help these tremendously traumatized parts begin to join outer reality. Some parts will always have been aware of what happened, but won't care to join the outside world.

Patience, allowing them to vent, will help most.

STEPS OF DISCIPLINE: STEP SEVEN: NOT CARING

This step will take the child further into a perpetrator role. The child will be forced to hurt others and prove their ability to not care during the process.

STEP EIGHT: TIME TRAVEL

The child will be taught spiritual principles of "traveling" both internally and externally, with set ups, role playing, and guided exercises reinforced with trauma. The goal will be to reach "enlightenment", an ecstatic state of dissociation reached after severe trauma.

STEPS NINE, TEN, ELEVEN

These will involve programming that will vary according to the child's future role in the cult. Sexual trauma, learning to dissociate and increase cognition, decrease feeling will be emphasized in these steps.

STEP TWELVE: "COMING OF AGE"

A ceremony of becoming at age twelve to thirteen, the child will be formally inducted into the cult and their adult role in a ceremony of "coming of age". They will prove this ability by performing the role/job they have been training for, to the satisfaction of the trainer and leaders; by undergoing a special induction ceremony. The ritual and ceremony will be held with other children of the same age, who are dressed in white and given a prize as acknowledgement that they have completed the basics of their training successfully.

They will continue to be abused, even as adults, but the major traumatization and creation of system templates will have occurred by this age. Future training will refine what was already placed in the child by this age, or build upon the foundation.

SUGGESTIONS

Grieving the abuse, acknowledging the feelings associated with undergoing the trauma will be important. It will be necessary to deal with perpetrator guilt, since by this time the child will be a perpetrator, and will have identified with the adult role models around them. This can be difficult to do, since perpetration will horrify the survivor when they remember this. Supporting the survivor, remaining non judgmental, and encouraging acceptance of these parts is important. Pointing out that at the time, they saw no other options available will help. Realizing that perpetrator alters saved the child's life, and that they had no other way to act, especially originally, the first time, will need to be pointed out. The survivor may feel hostile towards, or reviled by perpetrator alters, but they are the expression of the abuse and limited choices they were allowed. Grieving being a perpetrator will take time and caring support by others.

Lightning Source UK Ltd.
Milton Keynes UK
UKHW020658010520
362627UK00018B/1961

9 781911 417033